Function and Surgery of the Carotid and Vertebral Arteries

Function and Surgery of the Carotid and Vertebral Arteries

Ramon Berguer, MD, PhD
Frankel Professor of Vascular Surgery and Professor of Engineering
Samuel and Jean Frankel Cardiovascular Center
University of Michigan
Ann Arbor, Michigan

Illustrations by Lorie Gavulic

Wolters Kluwer | Lippincott Williams & Wilkins
Health
Philadelphia • Baltimore • New York • London
Buenos Aires • Hong Kong • Sydney • Tokyo

Acquisitions Editor: Keith Donnellan
Product Manager: Brendan Huffman
Production Project Manager: Alicia Jackson
Manufacturing Manager: Beth Welsh
Design Coordinator: Teresa Mallon
Production Service: Integra Software Services Pvt. Ltd.

Two Commerce Square
2001 Market Street
Philadelphia, PA 19103 USA
LWW.com

Printed in China

10 9 8 7 6 5 4 3 2 1

Library of Congress Cataloging-in-Publication Data

Berguer, Ramon, author.
Function and surgery of the carotid and vertebral arteries / Ramon Berguer; illustrations by Lorie Gavulic.
p. ; cm.
Includes bibliographical references.
ISBN 978-1-4511-9258-2
I. Title.
[DNLM: 1. Carotid Arteries—physiology. 2. Carotid Arteries—surgery. 3. Carotid Artery Diseases. 4. Carotid Artery Injuries. 5. Vertebral Artery—physiology. 6. Vertebral Artery—surgery. 7. Vertebral Artery Dissection. WG 595.C2]
RD598.6
617.4'13—dc23

2013028389

Care has been taken to confirm the accuracy of the information presented and to describe generally accepted practices. However, the authors, editors, and publisher are not responsible for errors or omissions or for any consequences from application of the information in this book and make no warranty, expressed or implied, with respect to the currency, completeness, or accuracy of the contents of the publication. Application of the information in a particular situation remains the professional responsibility of the practitioner.

The authors, editors, and publisher have exerted every effort to ensure that drug selection and dosage set forth in this text are in accordance with current recommendations and practice at the time of publication. However, in view of ongoing research, changes in government regulations, and the constant flow of information relating to drug therapy and drug reactions, the reader is urged to check the package insert for each drug for any change in indications and dosage and for added warnings and precautions. This is particularly important when the recommended agent is a new or infrequently employed drug.

Some drugs and medical devices presented in the publication have Food and Drug Administration (FDA) clearance for limited use in restricted research settings. It is the responsibility of the health care provider to ascertain the FDA status of each drug or device planned for use in their clinical practice.

To purchase additional copies of this book, call our customer service department at (800) 638-3030 or fax orders to (301) 223-2320. International customers should call (301) 223-2300.

Visit Lippincott Williams & Wilkins on the Internet at: LWW.com. Lippincott Williams & Wilkins customer service representatives are available from 8:30 am to 6:00 pm, EST.

FOREWORD

Surgery for extracranial vascular disease has been one of the most challenging disciplines in surgical history, exceeded only by coronary artery disease. Multiple prospective randomized trials have now proven the value of carotid endarterectomy (CEA) over medical management for both symptomatic and asymptomatic lesions. The latest challenge to the dominance of CEA has been carotid stent/angioplasty (CAS). We now have evidence from well-designed clinical trials in the United States, Europe, and other international participation which have shown that the complications of death and stroke following CAS are twice as high when compared to CEA.

Now that CEA has once again been established as the treatment of choice in carefully selected patients, this new text by Dr. Ramon Berguer is particularly timely. While this text follows a traditional organization when discussing a surgical discipline, there are several unique features that deserve recognition. First of all, the discussion of anatomy and particularly anatomic variation is a gem that will serve both the novice and the experienced vascular surgeon. I am not aware of any anatomy or surgical text that provides this detailed analysis. In fact, all of the anatomic variations that Dr. Berguer describes have come from his lifetime experience from which he has kept detailed record. This section alone is worth the reader's careful study. Likewise, the discussion of pathology is both succinct and comprehensive. Finally, the discussion of surgical technique that is beautifully illustrated reflects Dr. Berguer's mastery of his art over a rich lifetime experience. In addition to the technical discussion are sections that call attention to potential surgical error and how to avoid mishap, once again emphasizing the fact that while good surgical judgment comes with experience, we can all profit from the experience of those that share a lifetime experience with us.

In summary, this text represents a lifelong study, based upon a rich clinical experience that can benefit the reader, irrespective of their level of vascular surgical maturity. Reading this text was both a treat and an education for me as it will be for those who take the time to savor the information provided within.

Wesley S. Moore, MD
Los Angeles, California

PREFACE

I wrote this book at the tail end of a vascular practice that gave me the privilege of operating on a large number of patients with lesions of the supraaortic trunks and carotid and vertebral arteries. The narrative has a mechanistic bias because anatomy, the interaction between bone, tendon, and artery and the mechanics of blood flow and of the arterial wall make up a cogent story for the pathology of the carotid and vertebral arteries.

There are questions concerning indications, choice of technique, and management of complications for which a reliable answer will not be found in the many prospective trials available. In seeking answers to questions that have not yet been settled, we can rely on direct observation, understanding of the mechanisms involved, and accounting of outcomes. I refer to the sort of evidence that guides us to ligate a bleeding artery or to unplug an acutely obstructed one, without the guidance of a trial of observation versus intervention.

Vascular surgery is an empiric discipline that grew by trial and error. We use simple heuristics to deal with the enormous complexity of a diseased vascular system. Our discipline is, at its core, the skill to decide when and how to mend vessels. In what concerns surgical repairs, we want them to be simple and brief.

With endovascular procedures being a large part of the practice of vascular surgeons, operations on the arteries supplying the brain are less frequent and vascular residents, exposed to fewer procedures, may not have the opportunity of learning the maneuvers needed to resolve unusual situations.

The enthusiastic reporting from innovators and from industry-sponsored trials in the 1990s suggested that the open operations we had been performing for atheromatous lesions of the supraaortic trunks and carotid and vertebral arteries might soon be relegated to a distant second place by angioplasty and stent techniques. Eventually, well-designed trials such as CREST and ICSS showed that, in terms of death and stroke, carotid endarterectomy is safer than carotid stenting. There has been no clinical report of the outcomes of vertebral angioplasty in patients with vertebrobasilar ischemia and the long-term results of stents in the branches of the aortic arch compare unfavorably with those of their open surgical reconstruction. None of these considerations negate the fact that angioplasty and stenting may very well be the best option for patients with supraaortic or carotid lesions that have adverse local conditions, severe comorbidities, or short life expectancy. We recognize that the endovascular techniques brought elegant solutions to unusual problems that in the past required risky and difficult operations, such as repairing skull base aneurysms, arteriovenous fistulae of the distal vertebral artery, or internal carotid lesions in scarred or irradiated necks.

While the data available suggest that surgery is the best solution for most carotid and vertebral lesions, this proposition is valid only if we appreciate that not all operations done on carotid and vertebral arteries are the same thing, in the sense that an angioplasty may be quite similar to the next. When some multicenter studies report an incidence of surgical complications 10-fold greater than others, it can be inferred that the surgical treatment being provided is not of the same quality across all trials. Surgery of the ICA and VA permits no technical mistakes and, to keep the risk of death and stroke at the 1% level, the selection of patients needs to be continuously refined, the anatomic traps anticipated, and the technique flawless. For the last two reasons, I have expanded on any anatomic, geometric, or technical details I thought relevant to the safe surgical handling of these arteries.

With this book I want to share whatever wisdom I have gained through my surgical practice by examination of the errors I have committed. The reason for publishing it is to improve the benefits we offer our patients.

Ramon Berguer
Ann Arbor, Michigan

CONTENTS

ABBREVIATIONS

The following abbreviations are used throughout the text:

ACA	Anterior cerebral artery
APN	Accessory phrenic nerve
AV	Arteriovenous
BA	Basilar artery
CA	Carotid artery
CBT	Carotid body tumor
CCA	Common carotid artery
CEA	Carotid endarterectomy
CTA	Computerized tomography angiogram
ECA	External carotid artery
EJV	External jugular vein
FMD	Fibromuscular dysplasia
GSM	Gray scale median
IA	Innominate artery
ICA	Internal carotid artery
IJV	Internal jugular vein
Lt	Left
MCA	Middle cerebral artery
MR	Magnetic resonance
MRA	Magnetic resonance angiogram
MRI	Magnetic resonance image
PAt	Proatlantal artery
PCA	Posterior cerebral artery
PICA	Posterior–inferior cerebellar artery
PN	Phrenic nerve
Rt	Right
rSA	Retroesophageal subclavian artery
RSD	Reflex sympathetic dystrophy
SA	Subclavian artery
TIA	Transient ischemic attack
US	Ultrasound
VA	Vertebral artery
VBI	Vertebrobasilar ischemia

CHAPTER 1

Anatomy and Function of the Carotid and Vertebral Systems

THE BRANCHES OF THE AORTIC ARCH (SUPRAAORTIC TRUNKS)

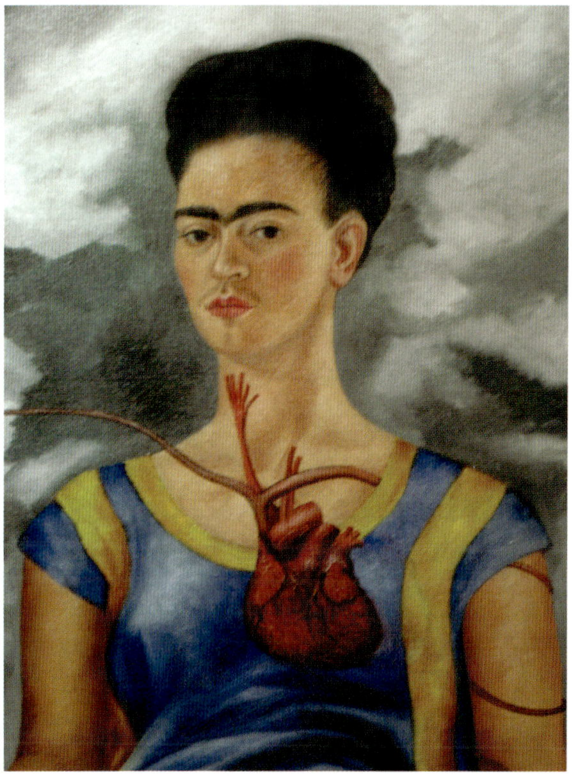

PLATE 1.1. Fragment of *Las Dos Fridas*, with Frieda Kahlo's (1907 to 1954) interpretation of the branches of the aortic arch.

Anatomy and Variations

The normal sequence (82%) for the takeoff of the branches of the aortic arch (Fig. 1.1) is for the innominate artery (IA) and left (Lt) common carotid artery (CCA) to exit first in the anterior mediastinum and for the Lt subclavian artery (SA) to arise from the distal arch in the posterior mediastinum. The distance between the origin of the Lt CCA and Lt SA (1 to 2 cm) is usually greater than that between the IA and the Lt CCA.

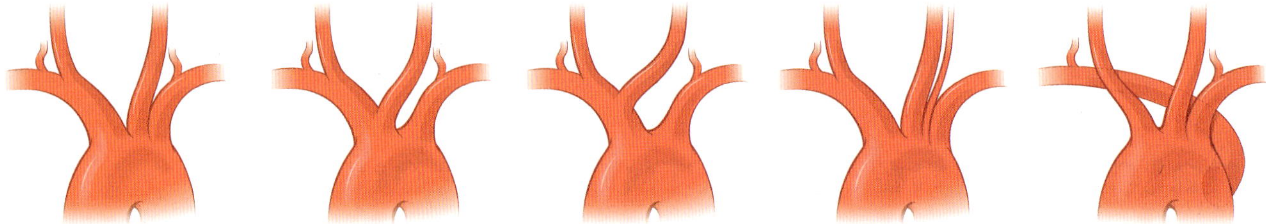

FIGURE 1.1. Variation in the origin of the supraaortic trunks.

The most common variation (10%) of the aortic arch branches is for the Lt CCA to take origin more proximally in the arch, either sharing the ostium with the IA or arising from the IA itself. The incidence of this variant is higher among blacks than in whites. This variant is relevant to the surgeon because clamping or doing an angioplasty of such a configuration will involve necessarily the blood supply to both hemispheres.

Another variation (10%) is a V-shaped origin of both CCAs from a single ostium, or from a short common bi-carotid trunk, before they separate to go to each side of the neck. This variation, present in patients who have an anomalous right (Rt) retroesophageal subclavian artery (rSA), is incorrectly designated as a "bovine" pattern.[1,i]

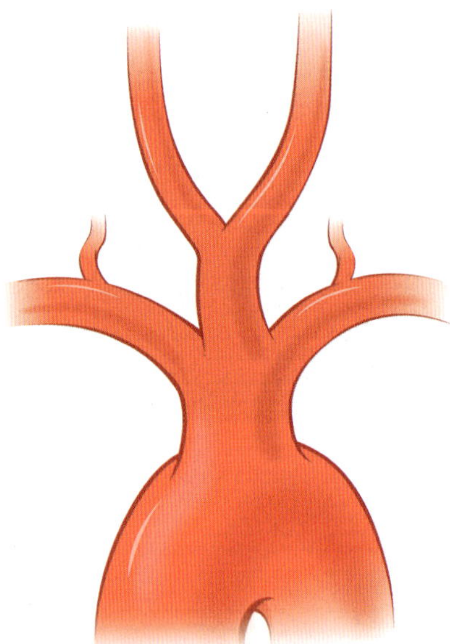

FIGURE 1.2. The aortic in arch in bovines.

[i] Layton has reminded us that this human variation is not similar to the arch branching pattern found in cattle (Fig. 1.2).

A third variation is the Lt vertebral artery (VA) arising from the aortic arch between the origins of the Lt SA and Lt CCA. This occurs in 7% of the people and, as we will see later (see Segment V1: The extraforaminal course p.19), this variation requires specific considerations during operations in the Lt SA and Lt VA.

When the IA takes off from the aorta more distally, to the left of the trachea, it must cross over the latter to reach its destination in the right side of the neck. The compression of the IA over the trachea results in different problems depending on which of the two elements is stiffer. Newborns with their soft, collapsible tracheas may experience severe respiratory distress if the IA compresses them. In most newborns, the IA, or some part of it, exits the arch of the aorta to the left of the trachea. By the age of 3 years, the growth of the aortic arch will have situated the origin of the IA to the right of the trachea and so it does not cross the latter. Babies with bouts of apnea or recurrent tracheobronchitis that do not respond to medical management will need surgical correction, usually transposition of the origin of the IA to a more proximal site in the arch. Conversely, patients that have a permanent tracheostomy cannula, or are undergoing long-term endotracheal intubation, may experience catastrophic bleeding when the posterior wall of the IA is eroded by the stiffened, cannulated trachea (aorto-IA fistula).

Clinical Implications of Aortic Arch Anomalies

A Rt rSA is present in 0.8% of the population (Fig. 1.1). Individuals with this anomalous artery have all or some of the following associated anomalies: a right-sided thoracic duct, a non-recurrent right inferior laryngeal nerve, and a common origin for both CCAs (Fig. 1.3). The Rt VA may arise in these patients from the Rt SA, the Rt CCA, or the IA.

The Rt rSA has an abnormal architecture and, like other persistent embryonic arteries (such as the sciatic, trigeminal, and so forth), has a propensity to degenerate early into atherosclerotic or aneurysmal disease. Aneurysms of the rSA can reach enormous size (Fig. 1.4) and may rupture into the esophagus. A Rt rSA may originate

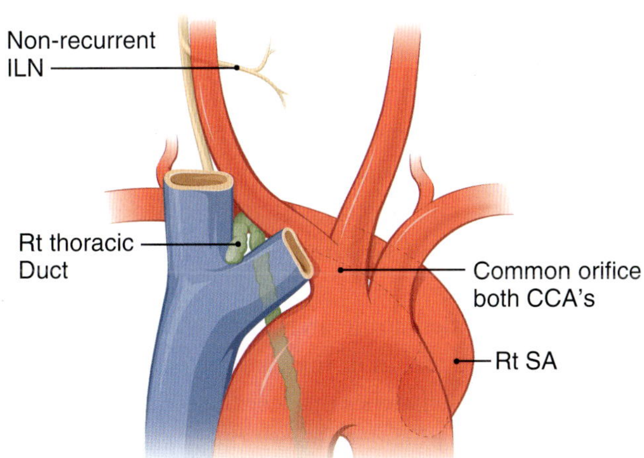

FIGURE 1.3. Developmental anomalies associated with a Rt rSA.

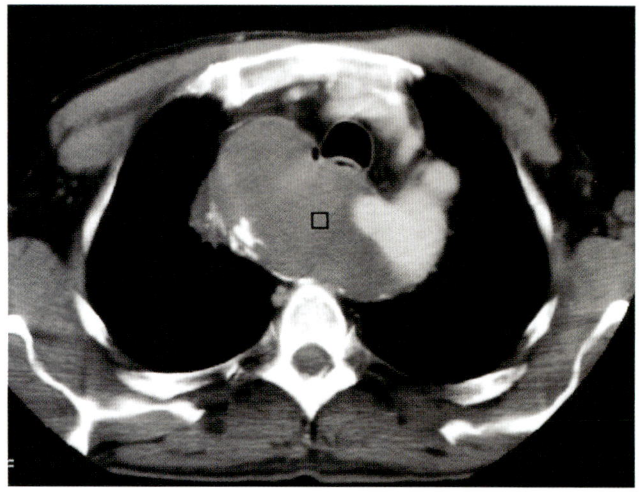

B

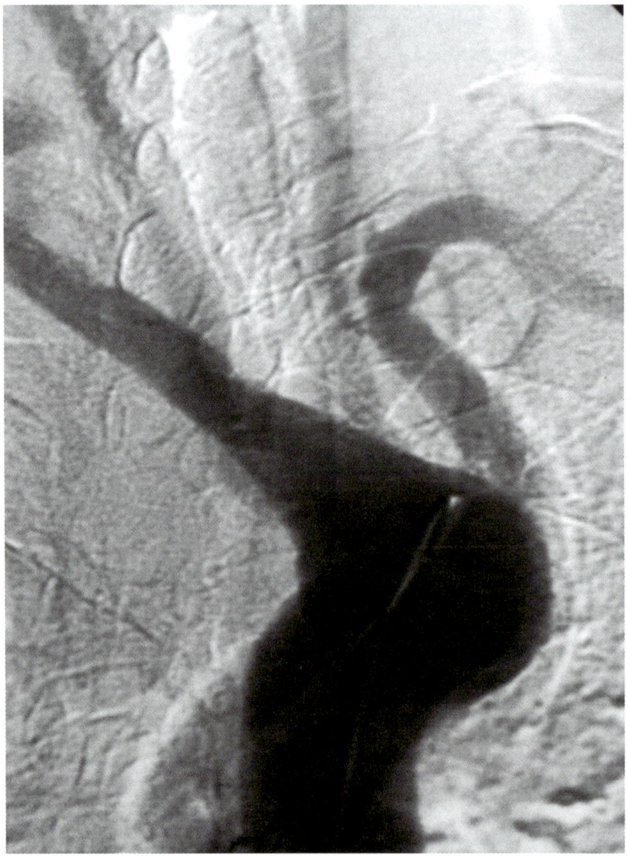

A

FIGURE 1.4. (**A**) Large aneurysm with (**B**) mural thrombus in a Rt rSA. The esophagus is compressed by the aneurysm.

from a normal appearing descending aorta or, more frequently, from an outpouching of the aortic wall called a diverticulum of Kommerell. The aortic wall around the opening of the Kommerell's diverticulum also has an abnormal structure and is often dilated above and below the opening of the diverticulum. This dilation may extend to the neighboring Lt SA (Fig. 1.5).

In a previous publication,[2] I had described the direct closure of the Kommerell diverticulum by an intralumenal patch sawn through an anterior aortotomy. This turned out to be a bad surgical solution. Over the years, patients show dilation of the aortic wall around the patch that closed the origin of the diverticulum. The current treatment of a diverticulum of Kommerell, covering its opening as well as the adjacent aortic wall with an endograft, is a far better solution, one that not only obliterates the opening of the diverticulum but also protects the neighboring aorta from further dilation. The coverage of the Kommerell opening is complemented by the transposition of the Rt SA to the Rt CCA through a supraclavicular approach.

Individuals with a right-sided aortic arch display mirror images of the arrangements seen in normal left-sided arches. If they have a retroesophageal artery, it would be the left one (Fig. 1.6). Rt-sided arches may coexist with agenesis of the Lt-sided IA (Fig. 1.7A) that will result in a Lt subclavian steal (Fig. 1.7B). A similar steal is present in patients with an isolated Lt SA that is not connected to the aorta (Fig. 1.8). Including the more frequent variations described above, a total of 25 different arrangements have been reported for the branches of the arch.

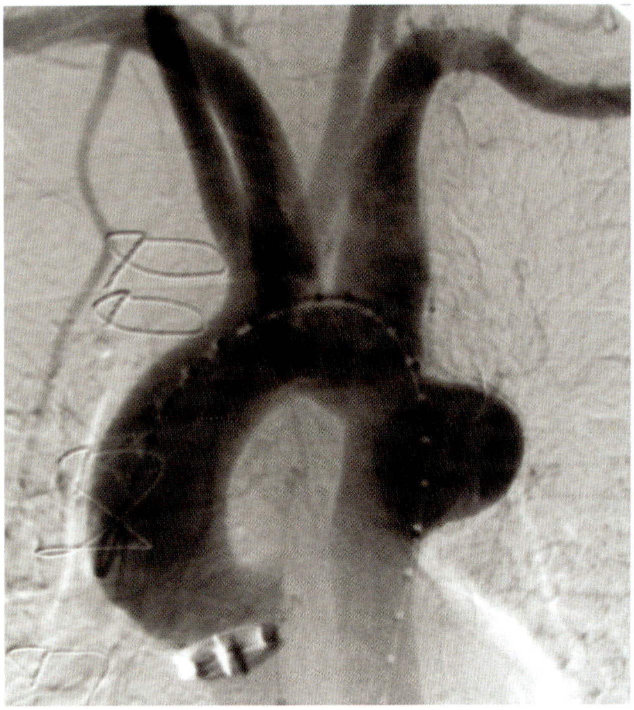

FIGURE 1.5. The dilation of the aortic wall surrounding the origin of the Rt rSA extends into the Lt SA.

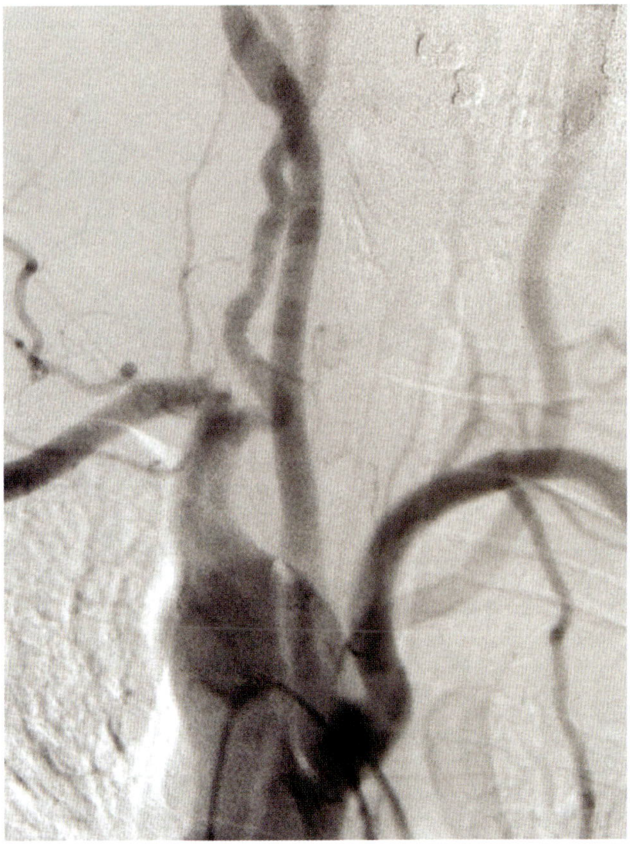

FIGURE 1.6. Rt-sided aortic arch with a Lt rSA.

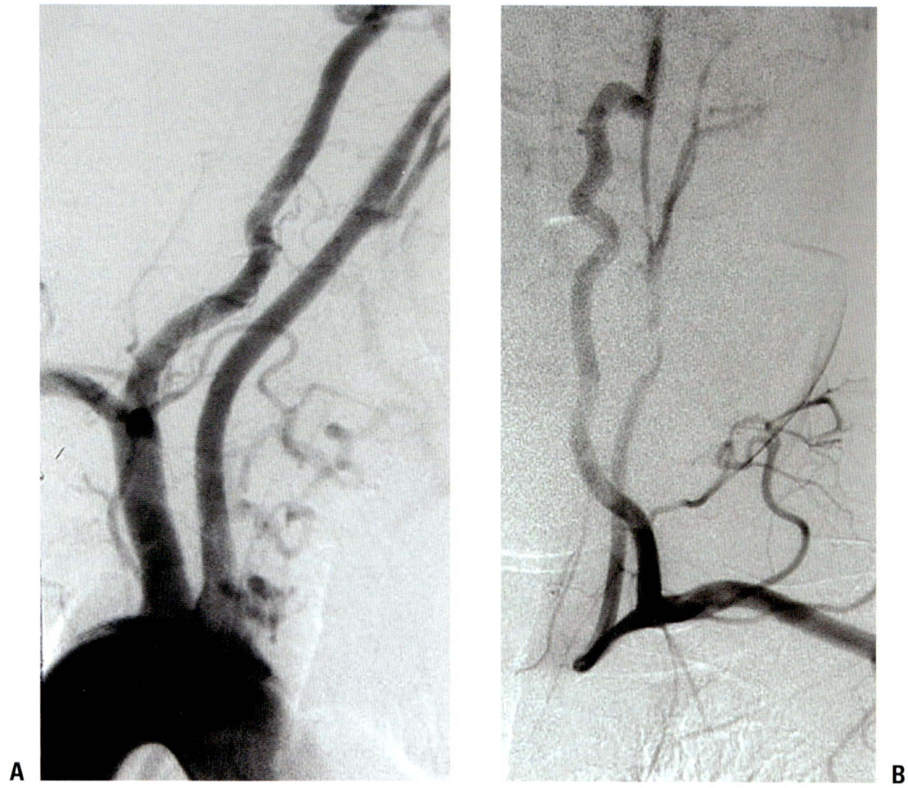

FIGURE 1.7. (**A**) Early injection phase of a Rt-sided arch with agenesis of the IA. (**B**) Late phase showing a vertebral and common carotid steal.

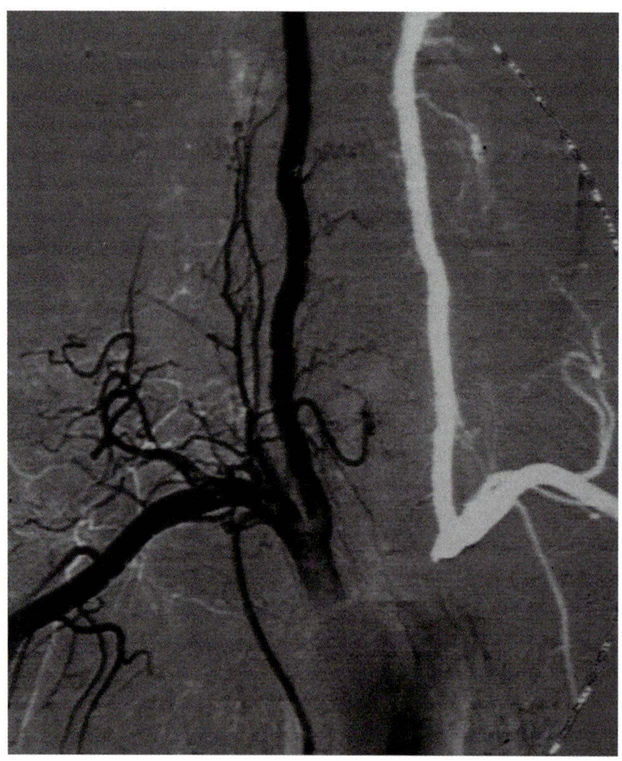

FIGURE 1.8. Subclavian vertebral steal in a patient with an isolated Lt SA.

The Phrenic Nerve and the Subclavian Artery

The following considerations regarding the anatomy of the phrenic and accessory phrenic nerves (aPNs) are pertinent to the finding of an elevated hemidiaphragm following operations on the SA. An aPN exists in 68% of individuals and its trajectory varies widely. An aPN may originate from the nerve to the subclavius muscle (containing fibers from C5 and C6) or from the ansa cervicalis.[3] aPNs are more frequent on the right side (Fig. 1.9) and 90% of them are lateral to the PN.

Injury to the PN or to the aPN results in paralysis of a hemidiaphragm. Injury to the aPN is one of the reasons for the surprisingly high incidence (between 10% and 85%) of hemidiaphragmatic palsy following cardiac surgery[ii] and for those cases where the palsy is found after subclavian venipuncture or supraclavicular nerve block.[4–6]

There are nerve loops around the subclavian vein and the internal mammary artery linking the PN and the aPN that may be injured during venipuncture and during high dissection of the internal mammary artery for coronary revascularization.

This variable topography of the aPN is the likely explanation for the finding of hemidiaphragmatic palsy following operations on the SA even when the integrity of the main PN was noted by the surgeon. The corollary is that any nerve that is seen joining the PN in the surgical field should be preserved.

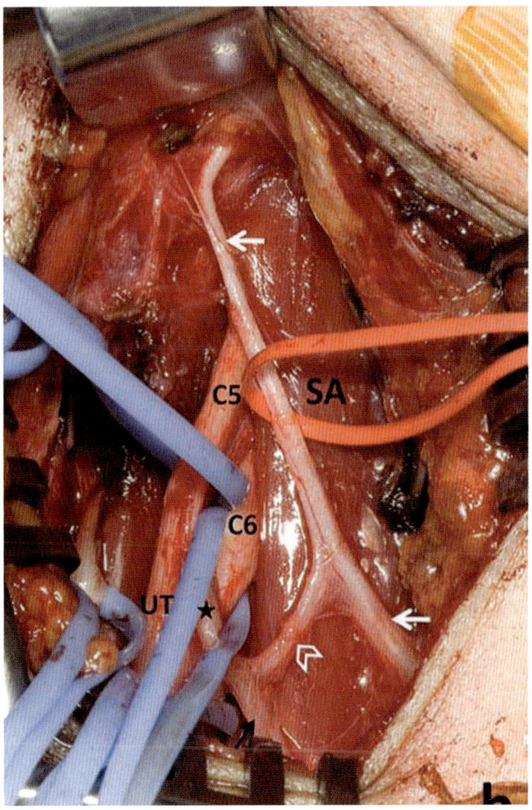

FIGURE 1.9. An aPN and its connection to the PN. Arrows point towards PN; Star (*) is on the aPN (With permission from Sharma MS, Loukas M, Spinner RJ. Accessory phrenic nerve: a rarely discussed common variation with clinical implications. *Clin Anat.* 2011;24:671–673.)

[ii] The other reason is cold-induced injury to the PN from myocardial protection strategies.

THE CAROTID ARTERY

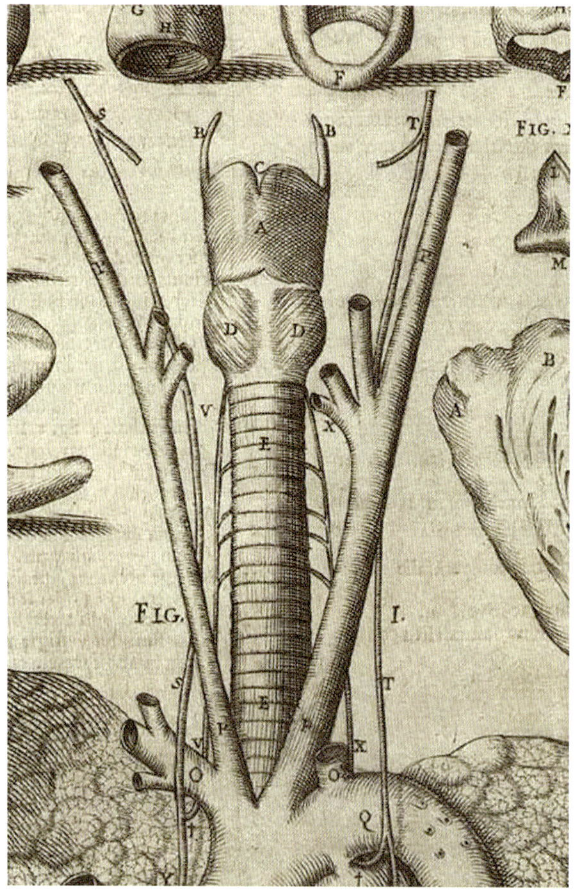

PLATE 1.2. Anatomy of the branches of the aortic arch. Fragment of a plate by Giulio Casseri (1552 to 1616). It is surprising that, until Boyd described the anatomy of the carotid bulb in 1937, this segmental dilation of the internal carotid artery was not depicted in the otherwise detailed anatomic drawings available in the XIX and XX centuries.

Trajectory and Histology

Arteries and veins do not have midline symmetry. The branches of the arch are asymmetric, the left and the right carotid may bifurcate at different levels, and carotid atheroma does not develop at the same rate bilaterally. The detailed layout of our blood vessels is not encoded in our genome[iii] but is believed to result from the interaction of vessel precursors with local factors.

The tortuosity of the CCA, internal carotid artery (ICA), and external carotid artery (ECA) has been attributed to age and hypertension although some observers that have noted ICA tortuosity in newborns have questioned this explanation. There is no denying, however, that the neck arteries we image in young people are straighter than those of older folks.

[iii] Identical twins have different venous patterns in the dorsum of their hands.

The CCA diameter increases with age and with atherosclerotic risk factors. As the CCA dilates with age, it must also elongate.[iv] Furthermore, the distance between the aortic arch and the skull base bridged by the CCA and ICA shortens with age due to shrinking of the intervertebral disks and increased lordosis of the cervical spine. The carotid arteries accommodate to this shorter distance by becoming tortuous.

Carotid coiling on the other hand (Fig. 1.10) is an embryological development and is not a consequence of vascular remodeling secondary to aging, hypertension, or atherosclerosis. Beigelman[7] showed in an extensive survey of 885 participants (from infants to nonagenarians) that coiling is not correlated with increasing age.

The carotid bifurcation is a junction of arteries with different mechanical properties the result of the different composition of their tunica media. The branches of the arch (IA, CCA, and SA) are *elastic* arteries. The CCA media is mostly elastin and collagen, as is the case with most conduction arteries. Conversely, the media of the ECA and ICA, both *muscular* arteries, is mostly smooth muscle with little elastin or collagen network. This gives the ECA and ICA the capacity to contract into spasm, as we see in the operating room when dissecting or stretching them.

The transition zone between the elastic CCA and the muscular ICA is at the origin of the ICA and extends distally for a length of 10 mm. The carotid baroreceptors,

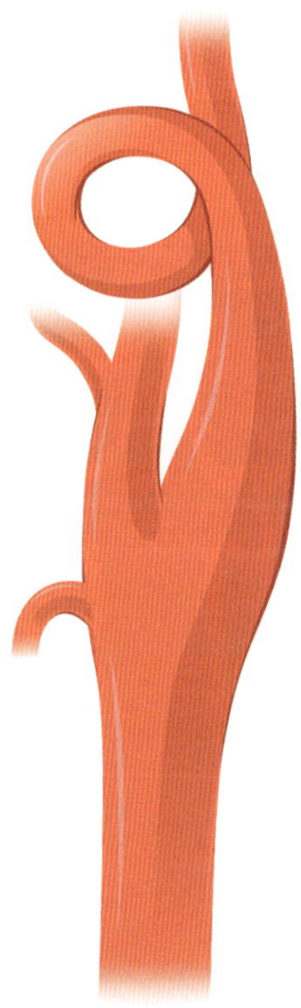

FIGURE 1.10. A carotid coil.

[iv] Just as a harvested saphenous vein graft increases in length when distended in preparation for bypass. Any elastic body that gets thinner (like the wall of an artery when it is dilated) must lengthen longitudinally. The Poisson ratio of a solid is the ratio of transverse to longitudinal strain. For the carotid artery this ratio is approximately 0.4.

located in this transitional zone, sense blood pressure by transducing their stretch. Most carotid atheromas develop in this transitional zone.

The bulb itself has a thick adventitia[8] (0.6 mm) and a thin media (0.2 mm) composed mostly of elastic fibers. At about 8 mm from the flow divider, the media doubles its thickness as layers of smooth muscle begin to appear. Sympathetic fibers run in the outer layer of the ICA and may be stretched and disrupted by the intramural hematoma of a dissection. This accounts for the high incidence (25% to 40%) of Horner's syndrome that is seen in patients with ICA dissection.

Internal Carotid Artery Aplasia

The entire ICA may be missing (agenesis) (Fig. 1.11) or there may be a normal size bulb and a thread-like or absent (aplasia) ICA distal to it. The opposite carotid or the VA that supply the territory of the absent ICA will be consequently hypertrophic.

Since the embryo's skull base develops 2 weeks after the ICA forms, patients with carotid aplasia do not have a carotid canal in the temporal bone (Fig. 1.12) and individuals with carotid hypoplasia have a correspondingly smaller carotid canal.

ICA aplasia (est. incidence 0.01%) is usually found in patients who are undergoing angiography for the workup of intracranial aneurysm: the incidence of intracranial aneurysm is 30% higher in patients who have a hypoplastic/aplastic ICA.[9]

The high incidence of intracranial aneurysm in patients with ICA aplasia has been attributed to (1) increased circulatory load in the contralateral ICA and basilar artery (BA)

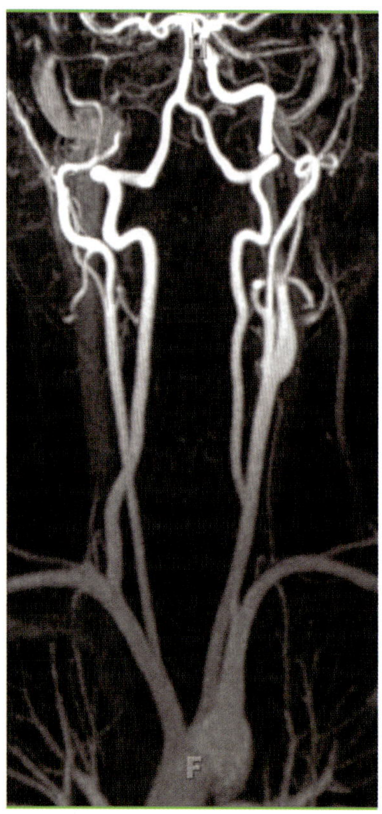

FIGURE 1.11. Agenesis of the Rt ICA.

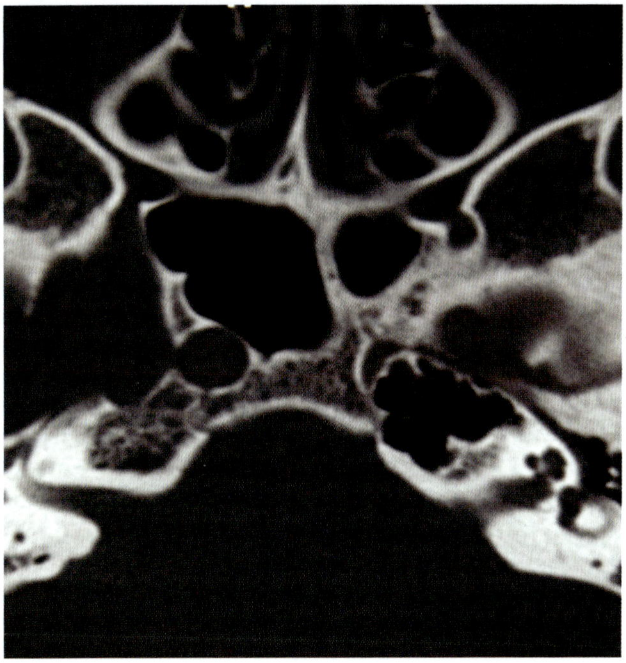

FIGURE 1.12. Absence of the Lt carotid canal in a patient with Lt carotid aplasia.

or (2) a synchronous error in development occurring at the fourth to fifth week of embryonic stage. But the fact that the associated intracranial aneurysms present more frequently on the same side as the aplastic ICA, in intracranial arteries that are not subjected to abnormally increased flow, makes the second explanation the likely one to be true. This explanation is further supported by the fact that patients with ICA aplasia often show other concurrent abnormalities (ventricular septal defect, hemangiomas) that are also believed to have occurred at about the same time (fourth to fifth week) that the ICA develops.

The Carotid Bifurcation

Carotid bifurcation atheroma is often asymmetric. Given that the arterial wall and its cellular components are exposed to the same humoral elements in both sides, it must be that differences in geometry determine the appearance of atheroma on one side or its absence on the other. The interaction of the flow stream with the geometry of the walls of the bifurcation determines wall shear stress, wall metabolism, the rate of local platelet aggregation, and factors that may enhance or inhibit the development of an atheromatous plaque. Because of this, some considerations are in order regarding the geometry of the bifurcation and what effects it has on these variables.

The CCA bifurcates at the same level only in 28% of individuals. The bifurcation is higher on the right side in 22% of individuals and in 50% is higher on the left. The CCA bifurcation may occur low in the neck, in rare cases as low as the upper mediastinum.

Measurements taken in the angiograms of a large cohort of patients show large inter- and intra-individual variation differences in the *geometry of the carotid bifurcation*.[10] The area ratio (β)[v] of the carotid bifurcation is 1.14 in newborns,[11]

[v] Ratio of cross-sectional area of ICA and ECA to that of CCA: $\beta = (A_{ICA} + A_{ECA})/A_{CCA}$.

remarkably close to the ideal area ratio (1.15) that the physics of flow predict for an ideal bifurcation that would minimize the development of pressure gradients and result in minimal wave reflection. The area ratio of the carotid bifurcation determines what pressure drops will take place as the single flow stream of the CCA branches out (ECA and ICA) and how much of the pressure wave will reflect and bounce back upstream. This area ratio of the carotid bifurcation may vary as much as fourfold between individuals. In addition, there is also considerable intra-individual variation in geometry between the right and left sides.[10]

The peculiar geometry of the carotid bifurcation, with the bulbous origin of the ICA, has been a subject of interest to those who study the relationship between the flow mechanics of the bifurcation and the tendency for development of atheroma in it. It is assumed that a lower wall shear stress on the sinus wall creates the physical conditions that enhance the risk of plaque development. Mathematical models suggest that the larger the angle formed by the bifurcation, the lower will be the shear stress on the sinus wall and hence the higher the risk of atheroma formation.[12] The bifurcation angle is larger in older people than in youngsters, perhaps a factor in the preferential development of atheroma in older individuals. Other studies using computational flow dynamics (with data derived from magnetic resonance [MR][13]) showed that some simple geometric features of the carotid bifurcation, such as the area ratio and degree of tortuosity, are good predictors of the site and rate of deposition of atheroma in the bifurcation. The numerical flow studies also show that turbulence and wall sheer stress gradients are greatly reduced when the origin of the ICA tapers its diameter gradually and does not have a bulbous dilatation,[14] which is, incidentally, the geometry achieved by a Type 1 eversion carotid endarterectomy (CEA), when some length of ICA is removed to correct preexisting elongation.

The first reference to the *bulbous dilatation of the first segment of the ICA* is from Allan Burns[15] who, in 1811, noted the presence of this dilatation "independently of any organic disease of the coats [of the artery]." Boyd[16] correctly concluded in 1937 that "changes in pressure of the general circulation are magnified at the dilatation and, consequently, the nerve-endings of the afferent nerves [in its wall] are able to register these changes in pressure more readily."

Physiology textbooks list the carotid bifurcation as one baroreceptor site, in addition to others that are presumed to exist in the arch of the aorta and its branches. These additional baroreceptor sites have been identified in some mammals, but Edwards[17] has reminded us that, in man, "the existence of arterial baroreceptors sites other than the carotid sinus, is inferred but not demonstrated."

If the carotid sinus is the only baroreceptor site in humans, it makes sense to preserve its function during CEA, particularly, when one considers that after endarterectomy we return the distensibility, the trigger for the stretch receptors, to a carotid wall that was previously internally splinted by plaque.[vi]

[vi] I have deliberately preserved the sinus during standard carotid endarterectomies. A frequent response observed was postoperative bradycardia and hypotension that could be reversed by 0.4 mg of atropine or by local infusion of xylocaine. The mild bradycardia and hypotension recede after the few hours that the baroreceptor needs to reset itself.

The Postbulbar Internal Carotid Artery

The diameter of the postbulbar ICA is smaller in women than in men, even after adjusting for body and neck size, age, and blood pressure. Toward the end of the bulb, the ICA is crossed by the hypoglossal nerve and further up by the digastric muscle. At about the level of the digastric, the glossopharyngeal nerve also crosses over the ICA and then runs beneath the ECA. At the point where it crosses the ICA, the glossopharyngeal nerve may not be a single trunk but rather one that has split into two different fascicles.

The ICA passes in front of the transverse process of C1 and is displaced forward by this process when the head is rotated to the opposite side. This mechanism has been implicated in the development of ICA dissection and the later formation of false aneurysm after motor vehicle accidents: as the head is rotated briskly the prominent transverse process of C1 moves forward striking the back wall of the ICA.

Further up the ICA passes medial to the styloid process and below the muscles that insert in it. The ICA enters the carotid canal in the temporal bone and at this level is separated from the middle ear by a thin bony wall. The artery leaves this canal to enter the cranium through the foramen lacerum where it perforates the dura and eventually traverses the sinus cavernosum. It finally turns upward and medially toward the clinoid process where it exits through the dura and becomes a short segment known as the supraclinoid ICA that eventually divides into the anterior and medial cerebral arteries. Important branches of the supraclinoid ICA are the ophthalmic, posterior communicating, and anterior choroidal arteries.

The *ophthalmic artery* supplies the eye and the structures of the orbit (Fig. 1.13). Two branches of the ophthalmic artery need to be considered when evaluating

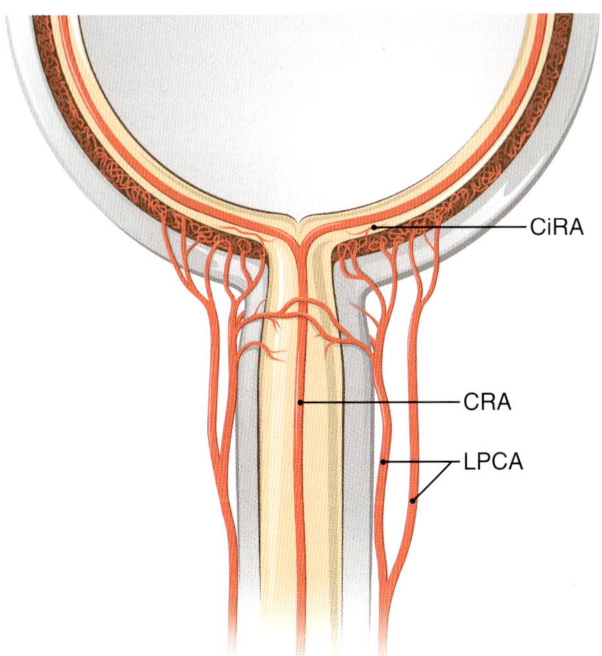

FIGURE 1.13. The ophthalmic artery and its branches to the eye. CRA, central retinal artery; LPCA, long posterior ciliary arteries; CiRA, cilioretinal artery.

ischemic eye symptoms: the central retinal artery and the ciliary arteries. The central retinal artery is a smaller vessel (0.3 mm diameter) and travels within the optic nerve to emerge in the optic disc as it divides into four quadrantal branches that supply the retina and can be seen through the ophthalmoscope. The posterior ciliary arteries are 0.5 mm in diameter and usually two or three in number.[18] They run parallel to the optic nerve and divide several times before reaching the eyeball as long and short posterior ciliary artery vessels that supply the choroid, the fovea, and specific sectors of the head of the optic nerve.[vii]

Occlusion of the posterior ciliary arteries may result in sectorial or total blindness by ischemic damage to the head of the optic nerve that they supply. In these patients, ophthalmoscopy will show the central retinal artery and its branches pulsating normally. The ciliary arteries can be assessed in magnified lateral orbital views of carotid angiograms.[19]

Cranial Nerves and Sympathetics in the Carotid Bifurcation Field

Four cranial nerves run close to the carotid bifurcation (Fig. 1.14). The **vagus** (X) lies in close proximity to the lateral wall of the CCA and ICA. The vagus is posterior or posterolateral to the carotid bifurcation in 96% of cases.

As the vagus descends with the CCA below the bifurcation, it rotates medially toward the anterior wall of the CCA. Here the vagus can be damaged when the surgeon extends proximally the exposure of the CCA in order to find a soft spot to place the clamp during endarterectomy.

At the level of C2 the vagus gives the **superior laryngeal nerve** that runs behind the carotid bulb and divides into an external and an internal branch. The external branch crosses the superior thyroid artery and eventually innervates the cricothyroid muscle and part of the pharyngeal plexus.

The topographical relation of this external branch of the superior laryngeal nerve to the origin of the superior thyroid artery is relevant to the vascular surgeon. In two-thirds of individuals, the external branch crosses the superior thyroid artery near its origin[20,21] and can be seen during isolation of the superior thyroid artery when dissecting the bifurcation. Injury to this external branch may result in the inability to project the voice, voice fatigue after extensive use, and decreased pitch range.

The **hypoglossal** (XII) nerve is usually covered by a large vein that drains into the internal jugular vein (IJV) above the facial vein. In high bifurcations, the facial vein will be the one covering the XII nerve. The surgeon must ensure that the hypoglossal nerve is not included in the ligature and division of these veins. Above and behind the XII nerve, there is a plexus of veins that runs parallel and close to it and the XII nerve may be injured when controlling venous bleeding at this level.

The XII nerve is often tented down by the occipital artery or by the sternomastoid branch of the latter. If this is the case when dissecting the ICA, dividing the occipital artery allows additional displacement of the hypoglossal nerve forward and

---

[vii] In 15% of patients, the posterior ciliary arteries also send a small cilioretinal branch that supplies a small patch of retina between the macula and the optic nerve. These patients may preserve some of their central vision even though they have occluded their central retinal artery.

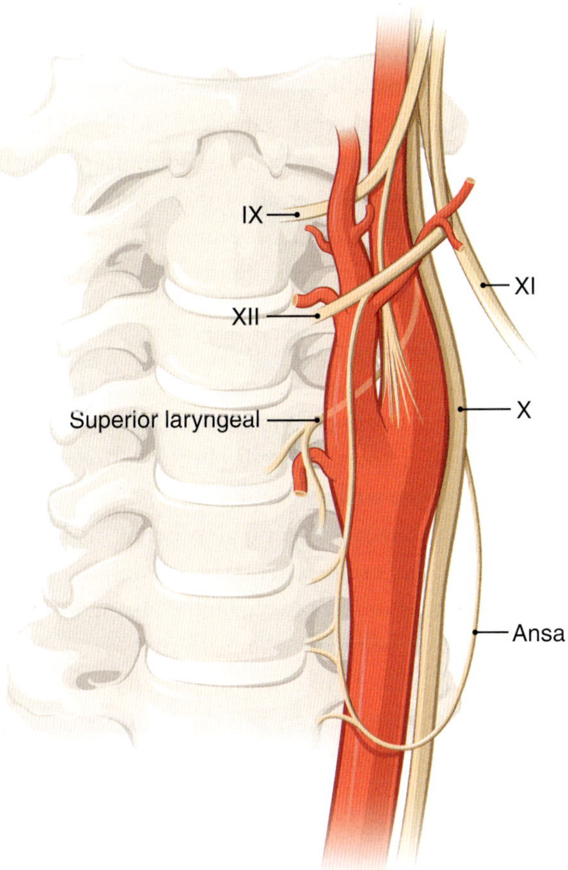

FIGURE 1.14. Cranial nerves in carotid field.

upward to uncover additional length of ICA. The **ansa cervicalis** is a branch of the XII nerve that links it with C1, C2, and C3, supplies the omohyoid and the sternohyoid muscles, and can be divided safely.

The **accessory spinal** (XI) nerve is found at 2.5 fingerbreadths from the mastoid tip between the anterior border of the SCM and the posterior wall of the IJV. It can be damaged during exposure of the carotid bifurcation if the IJV is dissected along its posterior border. The XI nerve does not come in close relation to the ICA until the C1 level where it rests on top of the IJV as they both cross over the (easily palpable) transverse process of C1.

The **glossopharyngeal** (IX) nerve courses above the hypoglossal nerve between the ECA and ICA. Trauma to this nerve results in a disabling swallowing problem that may require a percutaneous feeding gastrostomy. The **inter-carotid branch** of the glossopharyngeal nerve is the carrier of efferent fibers from the carotid sinus (baroreceptors) and from the carotid body (chemoreceptors). This inter-carotid contribution to the glossopharyngeal nerve travels into the brain with it.

A look-alike (sympathetic) non-recurrent nerve. When dissecting the carotid bifurcation one may encounter a nerve that seems to arise close to the vagus and wrap obliquely over the bifurcation directed toward the thyroid cartilage. Such a finding, when operating on the right side of the neck, brings to mind the possibility of it being a non-recurrent inferior laryngeal nerve. Unless the patient has a Rt rSA, the most likely identity of this "look-alike non-recurrent" nerve is that of an anastomosis between the superior or middle cervical ganglion and the inferior laryngeal nerve.[22] The way to resolve whether this is or not a non-recurrent inferior laryngeal nerve is to dissect it upward up to and beyond the vagus. If the nerve passes medial to the vagus into the deep tissues of the neck (toward the superior cervical ganglion) rather than arising from the vagus trunk itself, it is the anastomotic branch mentioned above and can be divided safely.

The **cervical sympathetic** chain runs from C2 to T1 over the longus colli muscle (Fig. 1.15) as a paramedian structure, 3–4 mm medial to the transverse processes. As they descend down the neck the two almost parallel chains converge slightly toward the midline. They are 56 mm apart at the level of the superior cervical ganglion and 45 mm apart at the level of the stellate ganglion.

Although classically the chain is described as being made of three ganglia, superior, medial, and inferior, this arrangement is seen only in 21% of patients.[23] The most common arrangement is to have two ganglia: a superior ganglion and a stellate (or cervicothoracic) ganglion below. A minority of 13% of the patients have four ganglia: superior, intermediate, vertebral, and stellate. The inferior thyroid artery runs transversely across the sympathetic chain and the latter fenestrates around the artery which passes through this sympathetic ring.

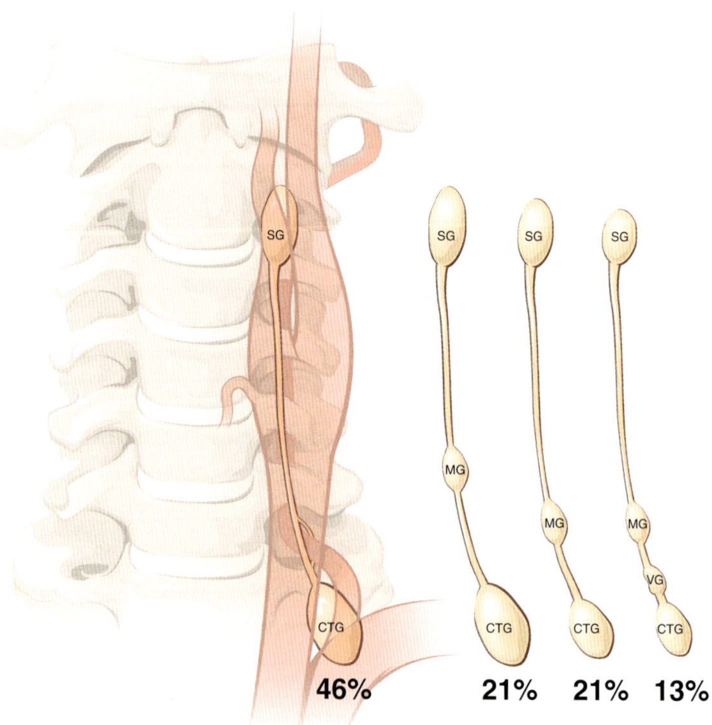

FIGURE 1.15. Sympathetic ganglia of the neck. SG, superior; MG, middle; VG, vertebral; CTG, cervicothoracic/stellate.

THE VERTEBRAL ARTERY

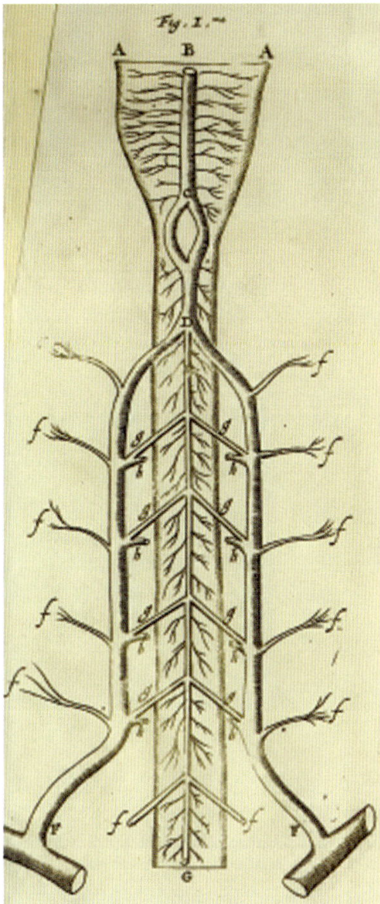

PLATE 1.3. The posterior circulation drawn by Willis (1621 to 1675). This accurate depiction of the vertebral artery supply to the spinal cord including the segmental contributions to the anterior spinal artery and the intervertebral connections appeared in his book *Cerebri Anatome*, published in 1664.

The Four Segments

The VA trajectory (Fig. 1.16) is conventionally divided into four segments*: V1: the extraforaminal* course, between its origin and its entrance in the transverse process of C6, covered in part by the accompanying single vertebral vein and by the intermediate cervical ganglion; *V2: the intraforaminal* course through the transverse processes of C6 to C2; *V3: the mobile* segment, from the top of C2 to the point of penetration of the dura at the foramen magnum; and *V4: the intracranial* segment ending in the BA. The anatomical layout of the VA is peculiar in that here two homologous arteries converge into one (BA) and, in its intraforaminal trajectory, the VA is attached to the periosteal walls of a mobile osteomuscular tunnel (see Chapter 2).

The VA is not, like the ICA, a branchless conduit. At each vertebral segment, the VA gives off radiculomedullary branches (Fig. 1.17) that contribute to the spinal cord supply, as well as osteomuscular and meningeal branches.

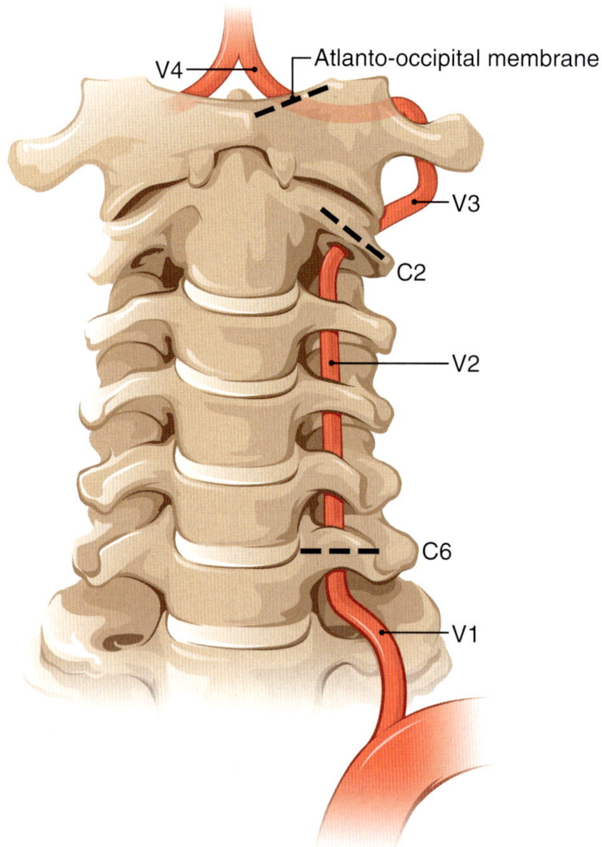

FIGURE 1.16. The four segments of VA.

The radiculomedullary branches anastomose, as arcuate arteries, with those of the opposite side linking, like the steps of a ladder, both VAs at each vertebral level. The VA can occlude segmentally and recanalize through one or several of these arcuate connections distal to the obstruction (Fig. 1.18). This is not the situation with the ICA that, lacking branches that could reenter blood flow beyond a blockage, occludes in its entire length.

Fenestration and Duplication of the Vertebral Artery

Although the terms "duplication" and "fenestration" are used interchangeably, they are meant to describe two different things (Fig. 1.19). In "duplication" one of the two arterial channels runs outside the vertebral canal. In "fenestration" the artery is a double-barreled tube with both components running parallel and close to each other through the same foramen transversarium.[24]

Duplication is common and fenestration is rare (Fig. 1.20). A special case of duplication is the double origin of the VA, often from two SA sites. The two VA segments join into a single VA trunk before entering C6. The clinical relevance of these duplications is in operations requiring placement of screws and plates in the spine, because the abnormal course of the duplicated VA could be in the path of a screw or a drill and be damaged.

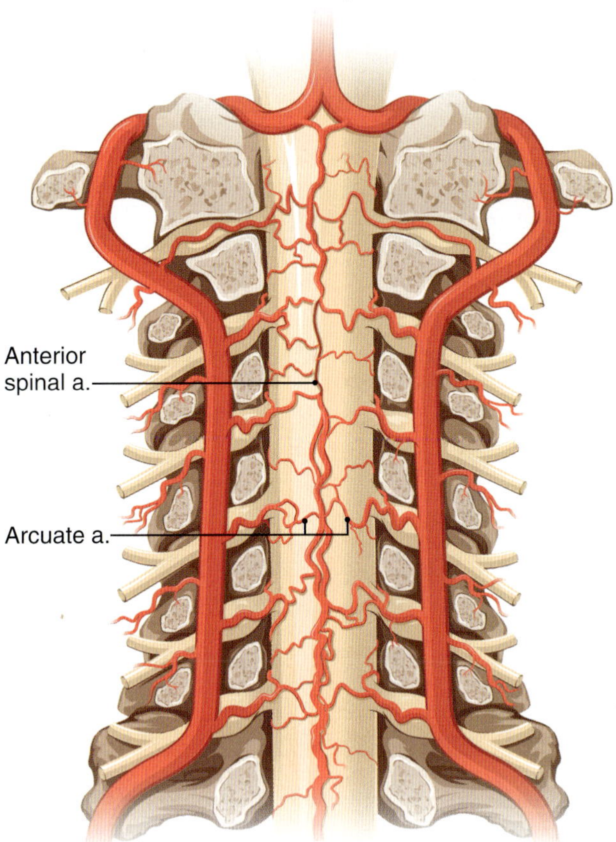

FIGURE 1.17. Ventral view. Radiculomedullary branches of the VA: an arcuate ladder between both VAs.

Segment V1: The Extraforaminal Course

The VA takes off from the posterosuperior wall of the SA. Occasionally, the origin of the VA is more proximal, in the mediastinum, within the first 2 cm of the SA. This latter pattern complicates the operation where the Lt SA is transposed to the Lt CCA in that the VA and the SA will need to be transposed separately to the CCA.

In 7% of patients, the Lt VA originates directly from the arch of the aorta between the Lt CCA and the Lt SA. When this is the case, the VA will enter the spine at a level higher than C6.

The vertebral vein is slightly larger than the VA and overlies it for most of its extraforaminal course (V1 segment). As the VA becomes tortuous with age, hypertension, and elevation of the aortic arch, it will meander away from the vein because the latter keeps a straight course. In this circumstance one may not find the artery behind the vein. The intermediate ganglion rests on top of the VA with rami extending medial and lateral to it (Fig. 1.21). Failure to preserve the integrity of this ganglion and its rami during exposure of the proximal VA will result in an incomplete Horner's syndrome (ptosis, myosis, but no anhidrosis) that may be temporary or permanent.

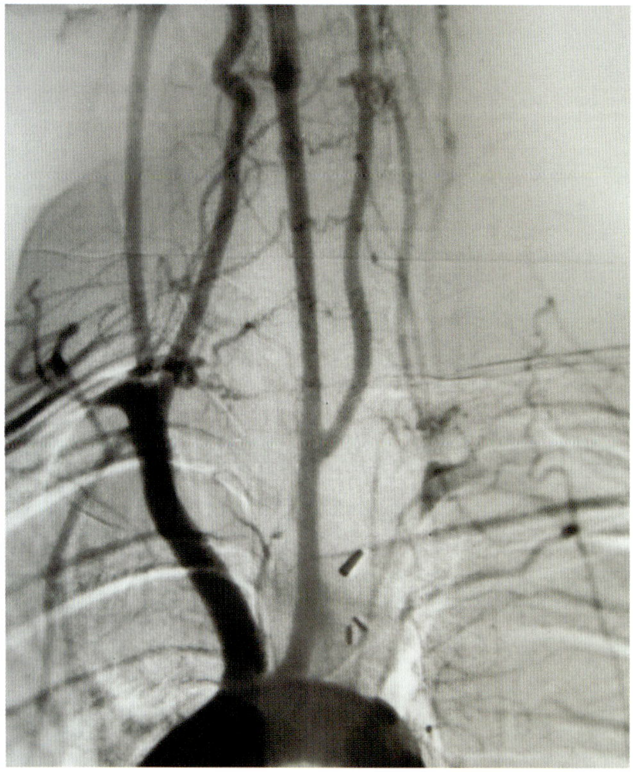

FIGURE 1.18. During childhood, this patient underwent repair of a coarctation with a SA flap that resulted years later in a large symptomatic vertebral steal. She underwent a transposition of the VA to the CCA. The dilated radiculomedullary branches linking both VAs that had contributed to the Rt to Lt vertebral steal are still visible in this arteriogram done after the VA transposition.

Before it enters the spine at C6, the VA passes under the musculotendinous slips of the longus colli and scalenus anticus muscles (Fig. 1.22). These muscle slips when contracted (contralateral neck rotation, abduction of arm) may compress the VA and arrest flow (Fig. 1.23). Compression of the VA by the tendon of the longus colli is more likely to occur when the VA enters the spine at a higher (C5, C4) level (Fig. 1.24), as it happens in patients whose Lt VA takes origin from the arch.

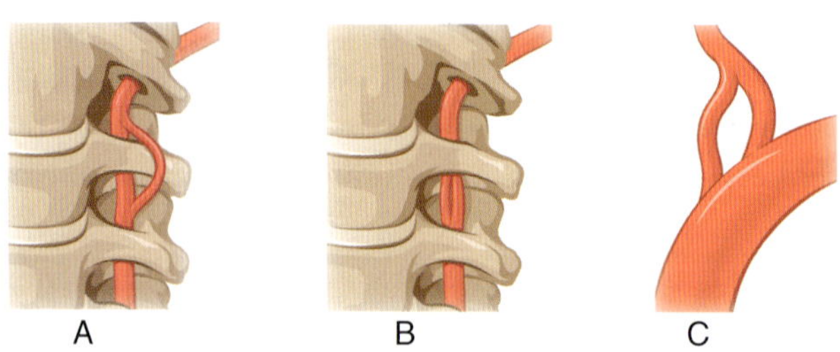

FIGURE 1.19. (**A**) Duplication, (**B**) fenestration, and (**C**) duplicated origin.

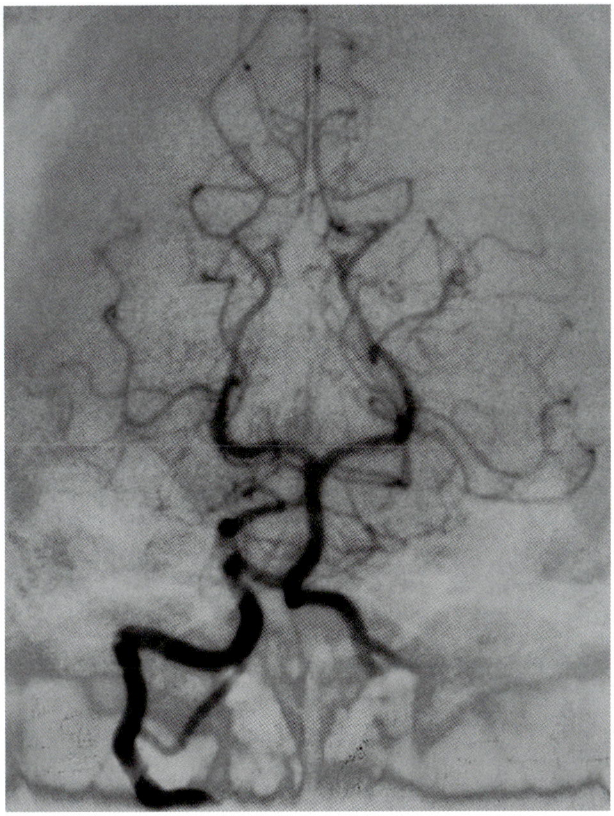

FIGURE 1.20. Duplication of the distal Rt VA.

Segment V2: Intraspinal Course. Transverse Foramina and Level of Entry of the Vertebral Artery into the Spine

The VA normally (95%) enters the spine at C6.[25] When it enters the spine at C5 (7%) or C4 (0.5%) it does so making a sharp turn into the spine (Fig. 1.22) and it is at this elbow that the VA may be compressed by the overlying longus colli or longus capitis muscles.

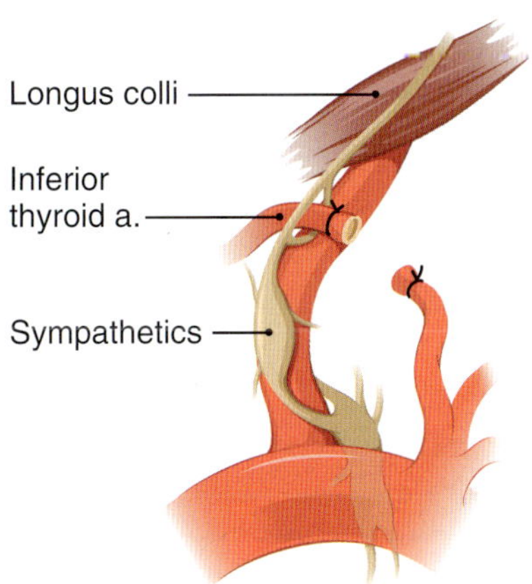

FIGURE 1.21. Relationship of the intermediate/vertebral ganglion to the VA.

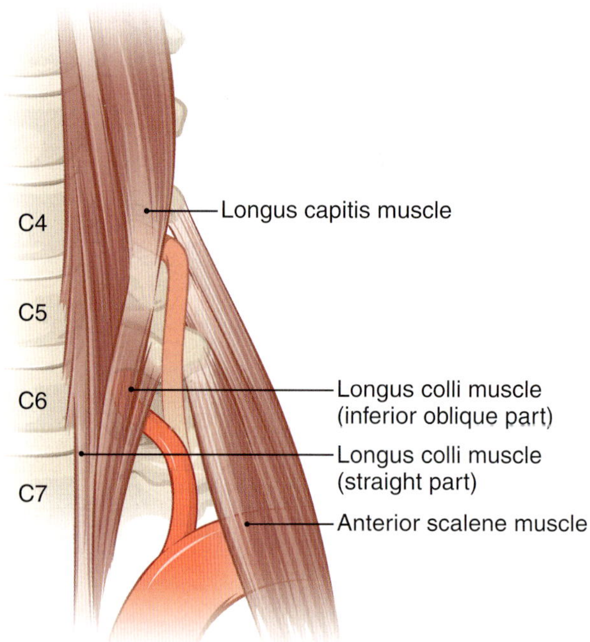

FIGURE 1.22. Before entering the spine, the VA passes under an inverted musculotendinous "V" formed by the longus colli and the scalenus anticus. The VA takes a sharper angulation as it enters the spine at a higher level.

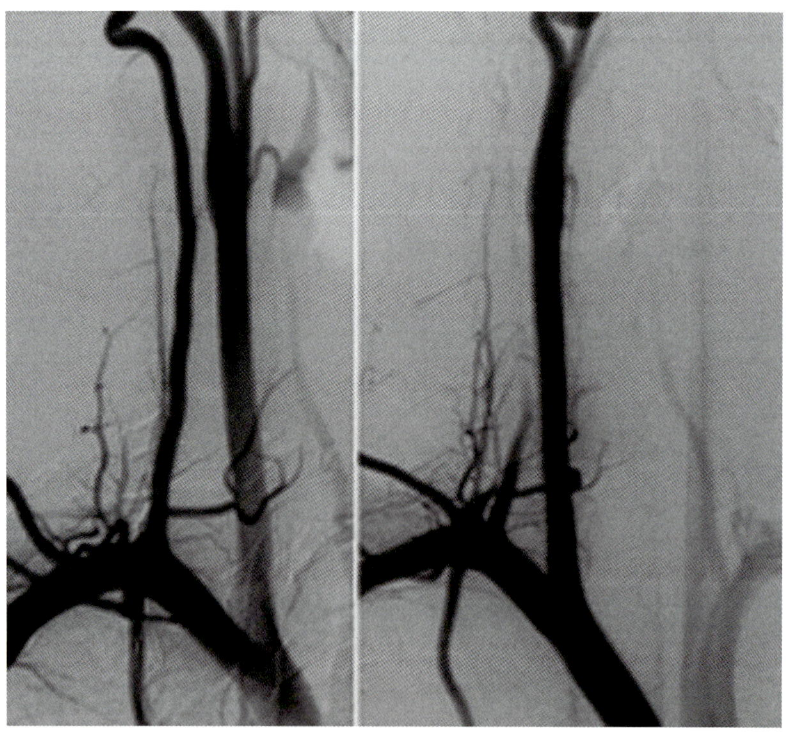

FIGURE 1.23. Compression of a dominant VA by the tendons of the longus colli and scalenus anticus during arm abduction. Lt, arm at rest; Rt, arm in abduction.

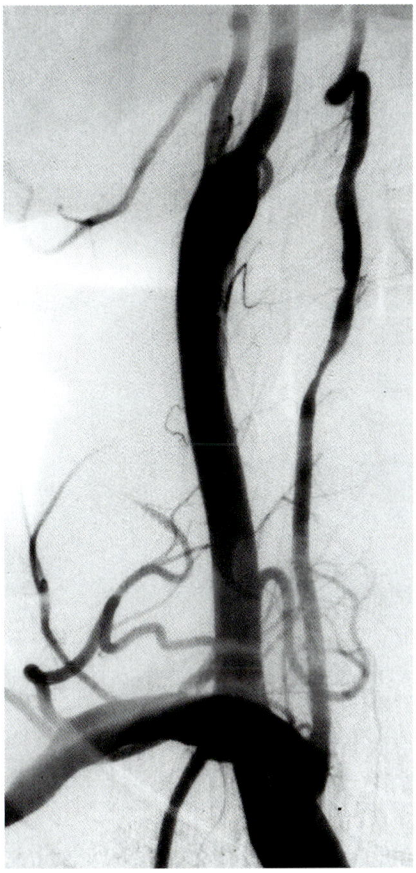

FIGURE 1.24. A VA entering the spine at C4 is compressed by the longus colli at this level.

A VA that enters the spine at C4 or C5 may be misinterpreted by a sonographer as being occluded proximally since there is no signal when interrogating its usual location between the transverse processes of C6 and C5. In 5% of cases, the VA may also enter the spine at a lower (C7) level and, when this is the case, the surgeon may have difficulty finding it. When the VA enters the spine at C7, it arises from the posteromedial wall of the SA and follows an almost horizontal course to the spine. Furthermore, once dissected, such VA will generally turn out to be too short to reach easily the CCA for a transposition.

In fenestrations, the double-barreled VA runs inside the transverse foramina; in duplications, the second artery courses outside the foramen. An extraforaminal course of the VA, whether the result of duplication or of an abnormal high entry into the spine, is of particular concern to the spine surgeon doing anterior cervical procedures, as it cannot be assumed that above C7 the VA is protected by the transverse process. An extraforaminal course for a duplicated VA is very rare, but it is worth remembering that whenever VA enters the spine at a level higher than C6 (incidence: 5%) the artery will have a short extraforaminal course over C5 and sometimes C4.

Throughout the V2 segment, in the space between each transverse process, the VA is accompanied by the vertebral venous plexus and rests posteriorly against the nerve roots (Fig. 1.25). This intimate relation of the VA to its venous plexus explains why arteriovenous (AV) fistulas develop so frequently after penetrating injuries of

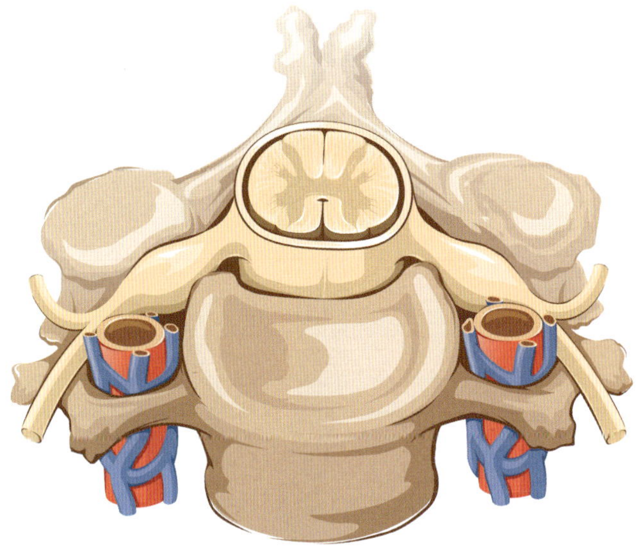

FIGURE 1.25. Relationship of the VA bone, vein, and nerve in its cervical trajectory.

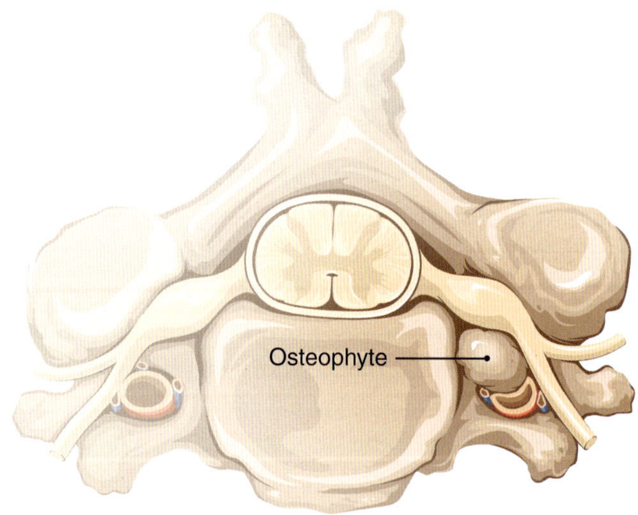

FIGURE 1.26. An oncovertebral osteophyte compressing the VA.

the VA. The VA crosses the uncovertebral joints at each level and the osteophytes that develop at these joints may compress and occlude the artery with neck rotation (Fig. 1.26).

The VA passes through the foramina of the cervical vertebras from C6 to C1. As can be expected from bone remodeling, when the VA becomes aneurysmal it will traverse a large foramen.[viii] In individuals with connective tissue disorders, when the VA becomes aneurysmal, the transverse foramen enlarges to accommodate the size of the

[viii] The earliest case of an extracranial aneurysm of the vertebral artery was described[26] in the skeleton of an adult male who lived in XV-century Gloucester, England, whose vertebrae showed gross enlargement of the transverse foramina.

dilated artery. The transverse foramen of the C7 that, normally, does not contain a vertebral artery or vein is smaller than the foramen of the rest of the cervical vertebrae.

Occasionally when *a VA fails to opacify in an arteriogram or computerized tomography angiogram (CTA)* there may be a question as to whether one is dealing with a severely hypoplastic or absent VA or with a VA that had normal size but underwent a dissection and eventually occluded. The size of the transverse foramena can resolve this question. If the absent artery had been of equivalent size to the opposite VA, their corresponding transverse foramena will be of similar size in the CTA. Finding a smaller transverse foramen on one side suggests that that VA was hypoplastic or absent. The area of the transverse foramina that contains a VA is larger, actually double, the area of those that do not.

If a VA enters the spine at an abnormally high level on one side, as is the case when the Lt VA originates from the arch, the transverse foramina proximal to the level of entry will be smaller than the corresponding foramina of the normal opposite side.[27]

Because the size of the foramen corresponds to the size of the VA that passes through it, the diameter of the transverse foramena decreases along with the diameter of the VA from C6 up to C3. It should be noted, however, that a foramen will develop in a transverse process even when the VA runs outside the vertebra without entering it. We see this situation in the patients mentioned above that have an abnormally high entrance of the VA in the cervical spine but nevertheless have a foramen in the transverse process of C6. It has also been described in the rare cases where the VA bypasses the C1 foramen before entering the dura.[28]

Vertebral osteophytes usually arise from the uncinate portion of the vertebrae that form part of the uncovertebral joints.[29] The uncus is only 1 mm away from the VA so that an osteoarthritic spur of the former may easily compress the VA (Fig. 1.27) and this compression will be accentuated by rotation of the cervical spine. Osteophytes arising from the zygapophyseal joints are less frequent.

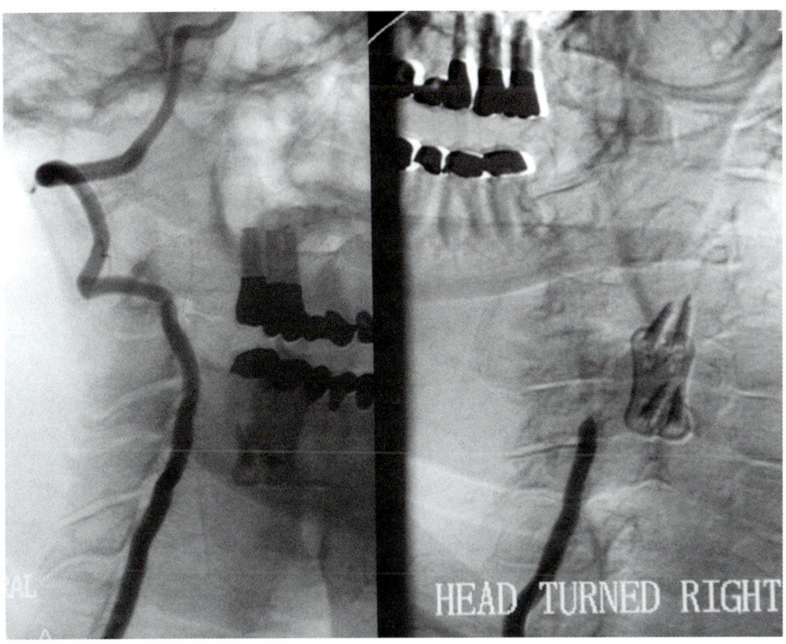

FIGURE 1.27. A dominant VA occludes when compressed by an osteophyte during neck rotation.

The **vertebral nerve** has been described as a distinct neural structure that accompanies the VA in the neck. Its function was not known and there has been plenty of speculation about it. This matter was settled by the work of Tubbs[30] that showed that this so-called nerve is simply a long and deep gray ramus that links the stellate ganglia to the C6 root.

The "Mobile" V3 Segment

The VA here has extra length to accommodate the wide rotational travels of the transverse processes of the atlas and axis to which it is attached (see Section "Dynamic Compression of the Vertebral Artery", p.57 in Chapter 3). The C1–C2 joint is the most mobile of the spine: one half of the entire range of rotation of the neck (180°) takes place between C1 and C2 (Fig. 1.28). The elongated loop of the VA between the transverse processes of C1 and C2 accommodates this wide arc of rotation.

The gap between the processes of C1 and C2 is larger than between any other vertebral level, a convenient help to the surgeon dissecting the distal VA in this location. After the VA emerges from the top of the transverse process of C1, it rests on a groove in the lamina of C1, the so-called pars atlantica of the VA (Fig. 1.29), before entering the foramen magnum. The groove is covered by the attachment of the atlanto-occipital membrane. When the lower edge of the latter is ossified, instead of a groove there will be an arcuate foramen or ponticulus ("little bridge") under which the VA passes (Fig. 1.30). In its trajectory over the lamina of C1, the VA may be compressed between the sharp upper edge of the lamina below and the occipital bone, above. If a ponticulus is present, the VA may be compressed against it during neck rotation. There are other abnormal pathways of the VA in its V3 segment (Fig. 1.31).[ix]

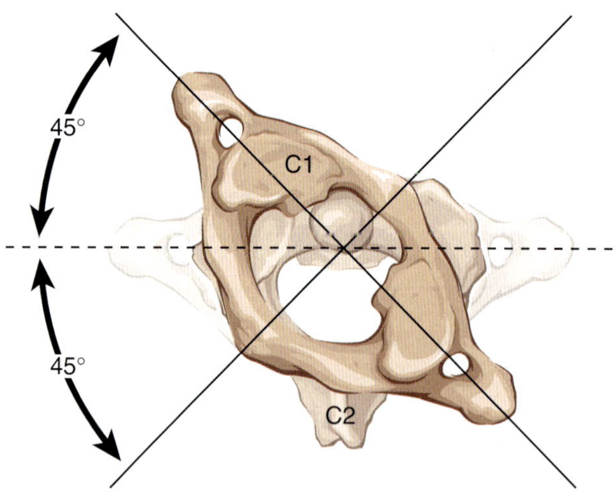

FIGURE 1.28. Arc of rotation of the C1–C2 joint.

[ix] Rare anomalies of this segment include an intraspinal course of the VA, avoiding C1 (a duplication) and a PICA arising from C2.

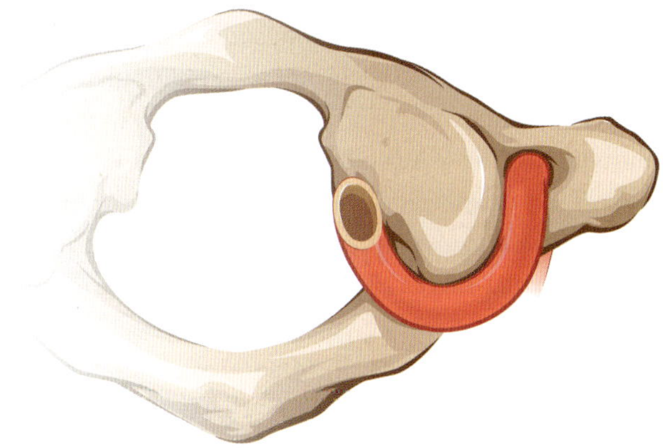

FIGURE 1.29. The *pars atlantica* of the VA on its groove over the lamina of C1.

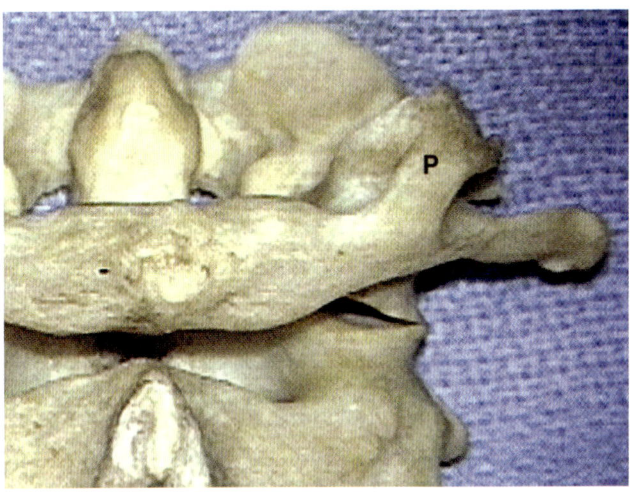

FIGURE 1.30. A ponticulus (P).

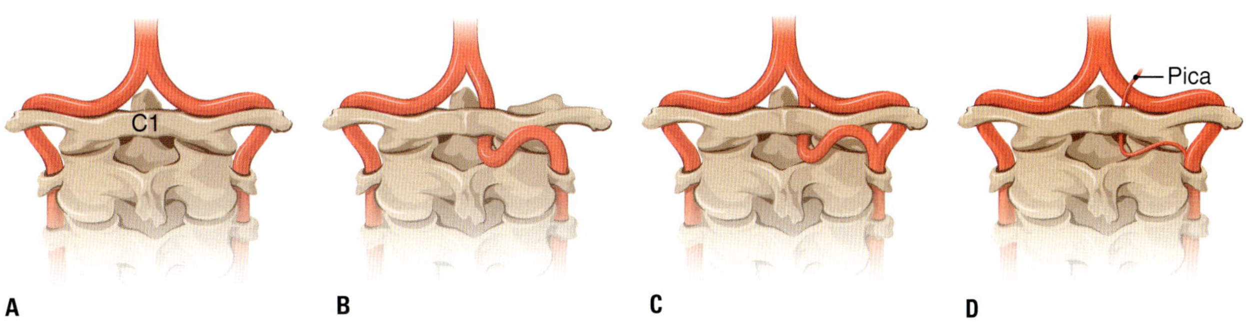

FIGURE 1.31. Variants of V3: (**A**) normal, (**B**) the VA avoids the transverse foramen of C1 and runs under its lamina, (**C**) duplication, and (**D**) PICA exits the VA above C2 and runs under lamina of C1.

The peculiar *biomechanics of the V3 segment* are at the core of distal VA pathology. In bow hunter syndrome, spontaneous dissection, sudden death infant syndrome and vertebrobasilar (VB) infarction following chiropractic manipulation, the thin-walled VA can be injured by being stretched between its attachments to highly mobile vertebrae.

In normal individuals, the VA is compressed at C1–C2 when the neck is rotated to the opposite side.[31] At this level, if the artery has been prestretched by neck rotation a rear impact force will cause rupture of the artery by adding further elongation to it. The inner layer (intima-media) will be the first to fail and the resulting tear may be the origin of a dissection. An even greater elongation will cause the wall to rupture creating an aneurysm or an AV fistula. In infants, the lateral mass of C1 is small and the atlanto-occipital joint is unstable. Coupling this with the large size of the foramen magnum, both VAs can be compressed and thrombosed in an infant[32] that sleeps prone (neck in extension) and rotates his head to clear the nose from the bedding.

The Intracranial V4 Segment

Part of this V4 segment is missing in hypoplastic VAs (5%) that end in the posterior–inferior cerebellar artery (PICA)[x] and do not join the opposite VA to form the BA. The wall of the VA in segment V4 is thin and has lost its external elastic membrane. Instrumentation of this wall with thombectomy or angioplasty balloons risks rupture and subarachnoid hemorrhage.

Dominance

Generally (85%) the VAs are not of the same size. When both VAs contribute to the BA, 63% show dominance toward one side (the left is dominant in approximately two-thirds of patients) and 35% show equivalence.[33] In the evaluation of patients with VBI secondary to low flow it is necessary to identify the dominant VA since this is the one that should be reconstructed. There is a relationship between the side of the dominant VA and the opening of the curvature of the BA as seen in an AP projection (Fig. 1.32): *the concavity of the BA opens toward the side of the dominant vertebral.* This configuration is already seen in newborns and is presumed to be the consequence of the unequal inertial forces of the flow streams of each VA acting on their point of convergence, where they form the BA, with the stronger flow displacing away the junction with the BA.[xi]

The flow patterns seen in this peculiar vertebrobasilar junction explain the frequent ipsilateral destination of emboli from the VA in the posterior cerebral artery (PCA) territory. There are two patterns of flow into the BA: (a) "parallel flow," seen in 80% of subjects, where the stream from each VA flow side by side through the BA without mixing and contributes preferentially to the ipsilateral PCA and (b) a "spiral flow," seen in 20% of subjects, where the streams rotate by more than 90 degrees from their entry site[34] as they advance through the BA.

---

[x] The PICA may exceptionally arise as low as C2 (Fig. 1.31D) and enter the spinal canal at C1–C2. This is a rare anatomic variation that should be kept in mind when doing a suboccipital approach to the VA.

[xi] A significantly higher percentage of pontine infarcts occur on the side away from which the BA is displaced, the infarcts probable being induced by stretching out the very thin, short perforating arteries that supply the pons.[33]

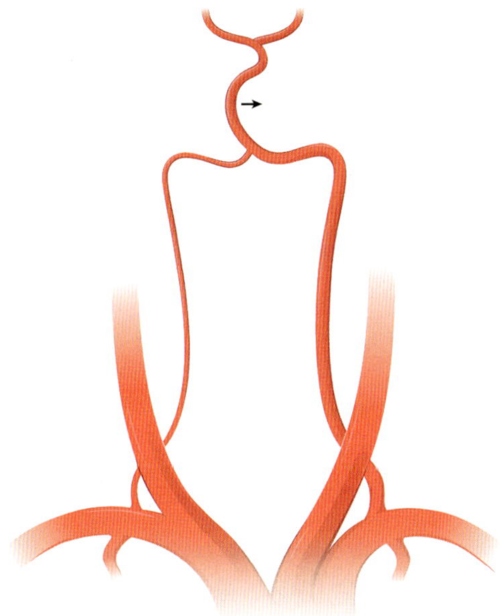

FIGURE 1.32. The concavity of the BA opens toward the side of the dominant VA.

Because the VA is enclosed into a tight and mobile osteomuscular tunnel, it experiences large changes in flow rates, even flow arrest, as the geometry of the tunnel changes with the movements of the neck. Weintraub[31] using MR imaging (MRI) and quantification of flow showed that head rotation consistently causes compression and occlusion of the contralateral VA at C0–C1 or C1–C2 level. In his study those patients who had a hypoplastic VA in the opposite side, and hence one that was not contributing to BA flow, were the most likely to develop symptoms during rotation of the neck (that compressed the single dominant VA). The demonstration of the occlusion of the VA during dynamic arteriography, synchronous with the appearance of symptoms, is essential for the diagnosis of symptomatic postural VA compression (see "Dynamic Compression of the Vertebral Artery", p.57 in Chapter 3).

The structure of the VA, like that of the ICA, changes as it enters the cranium.[35] As the VA penetrates the dura mater at the foramen magnum, it exchanges collagen fibers from its wall with the dura, anchoring itself to the latter.[36] The collagen fibers from the dura infiltrate the wall of the VA down to its media (Fig. 1.33). This explains why nearly all dissections of the distal cervical VA stop at the level of the dural crossing (the virtual plane of dissection is sealed by these radial collagen anchors that function like rivets across the media) and do not continue into the intracranial segment.

Throughout the cervical spine, and up to 1 cm before it penetrates the dura, the VA has a well-developed adventitia and a muscular media sandwiched between both elastic membranes. As the artery penetrates the dura mater, the media loses muscle, the external elastic lamina disappears, and the adventitia becomes devoid of elastic fibers.[35] In its intracranial segment, the VA is so delicate that it is translucent. This frail wall is probably the reason why the first trials of angioplasty of the VA in its intracranial segment were accompanied by a high incidence of rupture with subarachnoid hemorrhage.

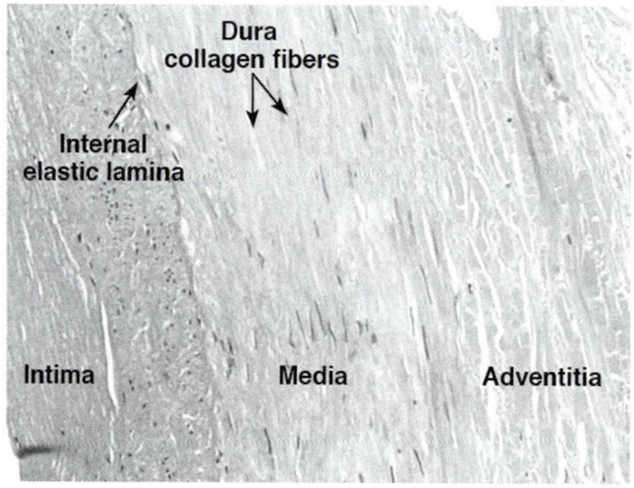

FIGURE 1.33. The VA wall is infiltrated by collagen anchors from the surrounding dura mater as it enters the foremen magnum. (Relabeled and printed with permission from Peltier J, Toussaint P, Deramond H, et al. The dural crossing of the vertebral artery. *Surg Radiol Anat.* 2003;25:305–310.)

THE CIRCLE OF WILLIS

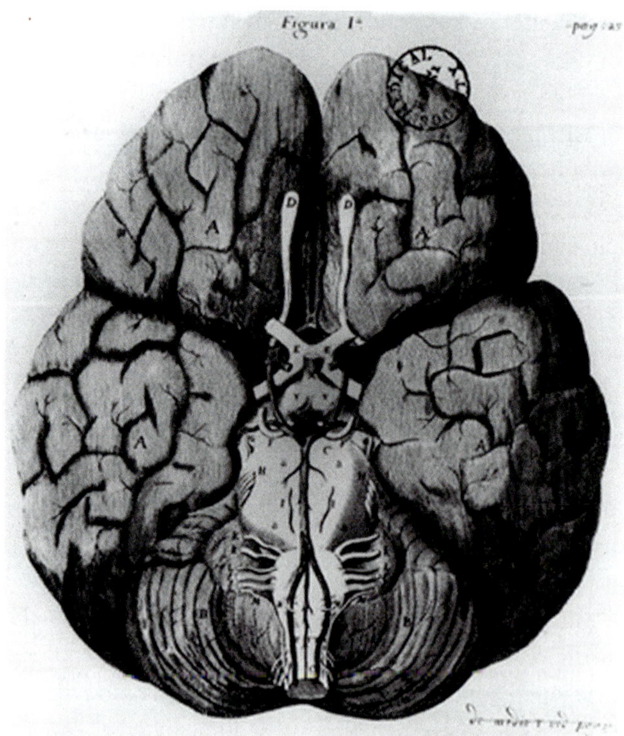

PLATE 1.4. The eponymous circle drawn on a copper plate by Willis friend, the architect Sir Christopher Wren (1632 to 1723). The drawing includes the Roman numeral notation for the cranial nerves devised by Willis that is still in use today.

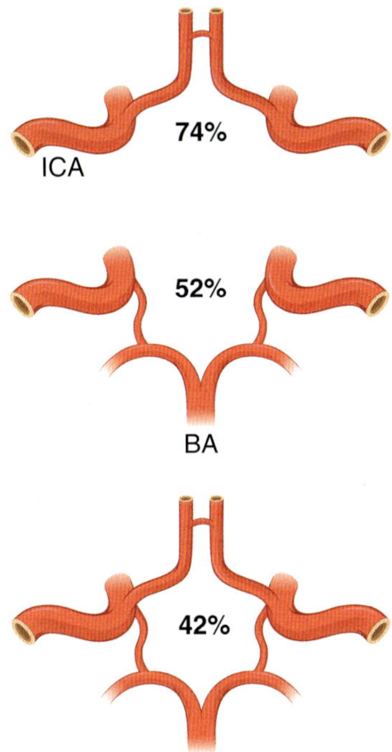

FIGURE 1.34. Incidence of completeness of the two halves of the circle of Willis.

A complete circle of Willis should compensate a flow deficit caused by any one of its three contributors: both ICAs and the BA. But a complete circle of Willis is present in less than 50% of the population and, in some cases, the size of the connecting components (anterior and posterior communicantes) may be insufficient to deliver the needed flow rate. Krabbe-Hartkamp[37] studied the morphologic variation of the circle of Willis using three-dimensional time of flight MR angiograms (MRAs). They analyzed the composition of the circle of Willis by considering its two halves (Fig. 1.34). The anterior half comprises the bifurcation of the ICA into the A1 segment of the anterior cerebral artery (ACA) and M1 segment of the middle cerebral artery (MCA), as well as the anterior communicating arteries. This anterior part of the circle was complete in 74% of the subjects. The posterior part of the circle is made up of the posterior communicating arteries and the precommunicating (P1) segment of the PCAs. This posterior circle was fully developed in 52% of the individuals. Only 42% of the individuals studied had a complete circle of Willis.

PERSISTENT FETAL CAROTID–VERTEBRAL ANASTOMOSIS

In the 30-day embryo, three, perhaps four, fetal arteries supply blood from the carotid system to the precursors of the BA (Fig. 1.35). When these arteries fail to regress, they will be present in the adult brain connecting the carotid system to the BA. These persistent arteries are often associated with other intracranial abnormalities or cranial nerve compression symptoms.[38]

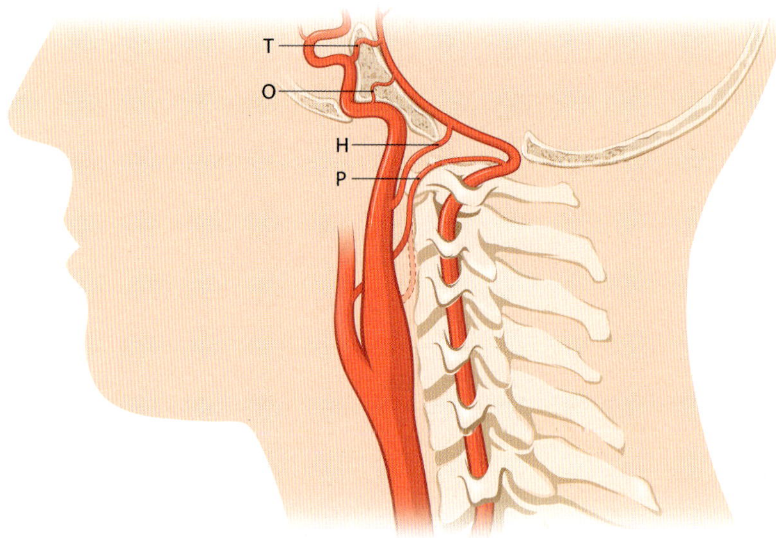

FIGURE 1.35. Schematic of the persistent fetal carotid–vertebrobasilar arterial connections. T, trigeminal; O, otic; H, hypoglossal; P, proatlantal.

The most common remnant of these fetal carotid–vertebrobasilar connections (85% of them) is a *trigeminal* artery that links the cavernous ICA to the BA (Fig. 1.36). When a trigeminal artery is present, the corresponding VA and posterior communicating arteries will be hypoplastic or absent.

The next most common persistent fetal connection is the *hypoglossal* artery (Fig. 1.37) that arises from the ICA and enters the skull with the hypoglossal nerve through the condyloid foramen.

A *proatlantal* artery (PAt) (Fig. 1.38) is a rare finding.[xii] There have been six angiographic demonstrations published.[39] When present, a proatlantal may arise from either the ECA or ICA and enter the skull through the foramen magnum as it follows the vertebral artery.

The aortic artery, which some authors believe may just be a low-lying trigeminal artery, is extremely rare and its existence is quite irrelevant to clinical practice.

[xii] I found a PAt in two patients during their workup for symptoms of cerebral ischemia: one patient had symptomatic carotid disease unrelated to the presence of the PAt. The latter had to be controlled with a Heifitz microclamp during endarterectomy as it was taking origin from the ICA bulb. The second patient presented with bouts of vertebrobasilar ischemia: he had developed a severe lesion in his PAt that was the only supply to the BA (both cervical vertebral arteries were absent). He underwent a patch angioplasty of this PAt (Fig. 1.39).

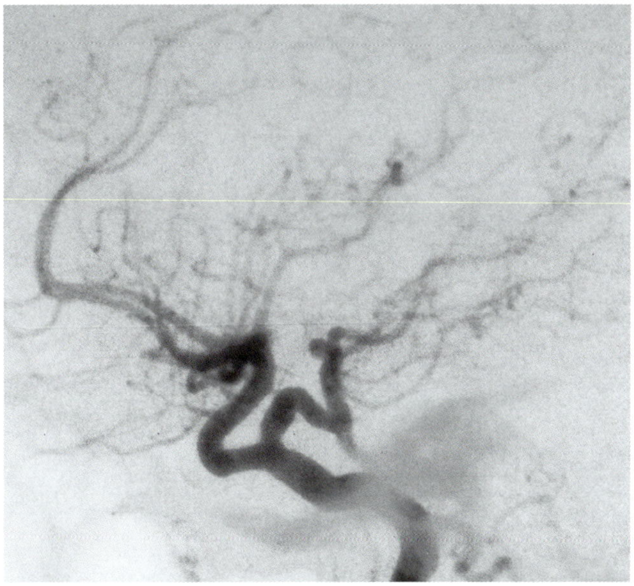

FIGURE 1.36. A trigeminal artery.

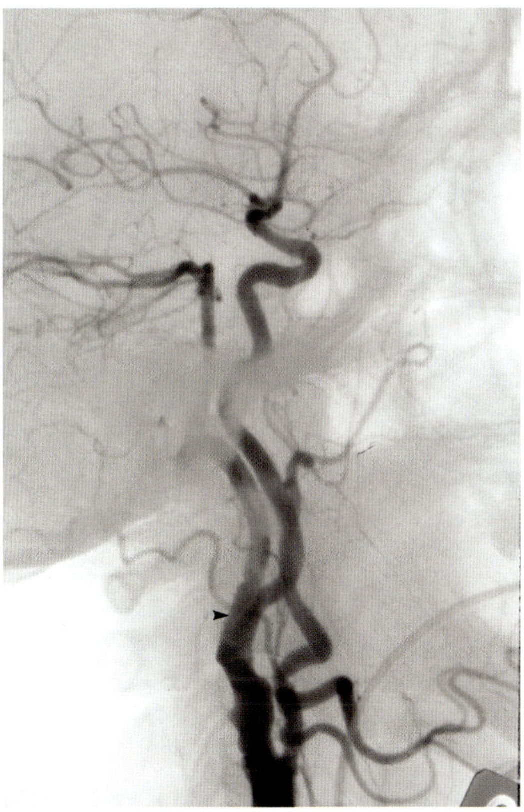

FIGURE 1.37. A hypoglossal artery.

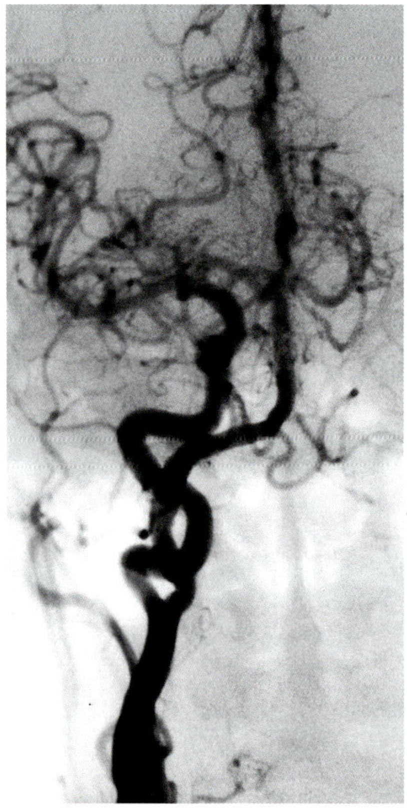

FIGURE 1.38. PAt supplying the BA and its branches.

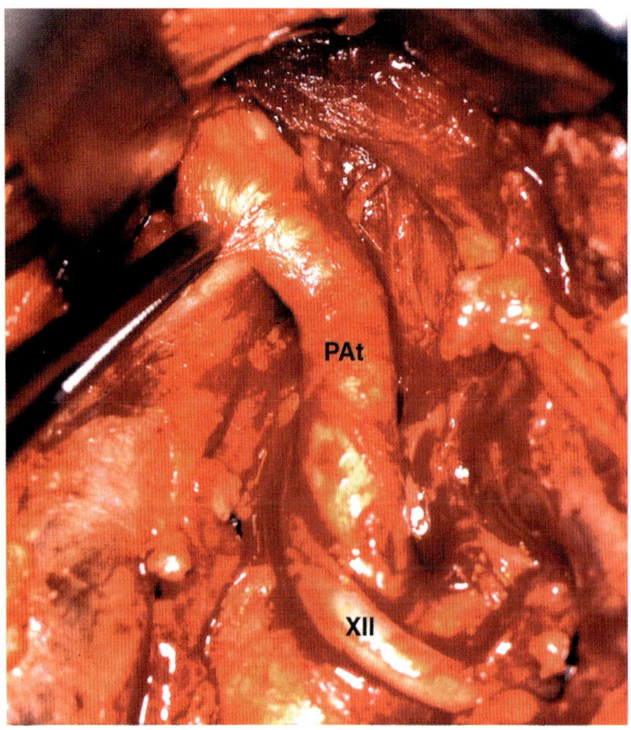

FIGURE 1.39. PAt looping over the hypoglossal nerve (XII) as it courses toward C1–C2.

REFERENCES

1. Layton KF, Kallmes DF, Cloft HJ, Lindell EP, Cox VS. Bovine aortic arch variant in humans: clarification of a common misnomer. *AJNR Am J Neuroradiol.* 2006;27:1541–1542.
2. Berguer R. *Surgery of the Arteries to the Head.* Berlin: Springer-Verlag; 1992.
3. Loukas M, Kinsella CR Jr, Louis RG Jr, Gandhi S, Curry B. Surgical anatomy of the accessory phrenic nerve. *Ann Thorac Surg.* 2006;82:1870–1875.
4. Tripp HF, Bolton JW. Phrenic nerve injury following cardiac surgery: a review. *J Card Surg.* 1998;13:218–223.
5. DeVita MA, Robinson LR, Rehder J, Hattler B, Cohen C. Incidence and natural history of phrenic neuropathy occurring during open heart surgery. *Chest.* 1993;103:850–856.
6. Sharma MS, Loukas M, Spinner RJ. Accessory phrenic nerve: a rarely discussed common variation with clinical implications. *Clin Anat.* 2011;24:671–673.
7. Beigelman R, Izaguirre AM, Robles M, Grana DR, Ambrosio G, Milei J. Are kinking and coiling of carotid artery congenital or acquired? *Angiology.* 2010;61:107–112.
8. Meyerson SB, Hall JL, Hunt WE. Intramural neural elements in components of the carotid bifurcation. A histological basis for differential function. *J Neurosurg.* 1971;34:209–221.
9. Lee JH, Oh CW, Lee SH, Han DH. Aplasia of the internal carotid artery. *Acta Neurochir (Wien).* 2003;145:117–125; discussion 125.
10. Schulz UG, Rothwell PM. Major variation in carotid bifurcation anatomy: a possible risk factor for plaque development? *Stroke.* 2001;32:2522–2529.
11. Sehirli US, Yalin A, Tulay CM, Cakmak YO, Gurdal E. The diameters of common carotid artery and its branches in newborns. *Surg Radiol Anat.* 2005;27:292–296.
12. Nguyen KT, Clark CD, Chancellor TJ, Papavassiliou DV. Carotid geometry effects on blood flow and on risk for vascular disease. *J Biomech.* 2008;41:11–19.
13. Lee S-W, Antiga L, Spence JD, Steinman DA. Geometry of the carotid bifurcation predicts its exposure to disturbed flow. *Stroke.* 2008;39:2341–2347.
14. Wells DR, Archie JP Jr, Kleinstreuer C. Effect of carotid artery geometry on the magnitude and distribution of wall shear stress gradients. *J Vasc Surg.* 1996;23:667–678.
15. Adams WE. *The Comparative Morphology of the Carotid Body and Carotid Sinus.* Springfield, IL: Thomas; 1958.
16. Boyd J. Observations on the human carotid sinus and its nerve supply. *Anat Auz.* 1937;8:386.
17. Edwards EA. Advances in gross anatomy in the 20th century. *JAMA.* 1977;237:1954–1959.
18. Hayreh SS. Posterior ciliary artery circulation in health and disease: the Weisenfeld lecture. *Invest Ophthalmol Vis Sci.* 2004;45:749–757, 748.
19. Berguer R. Idiopathic ischemic syndromes of the retina and optic nerve and their carotid origin. *J Vasc Surg.* 1985;2:649–653.
20. Kierner AC, Aigner M, Burian M. The external branch of the superior laryngeal nerve: its topographical anatomy as related to surgery of the neck. *Arch Otolaryngol Head Neck Surg.* 1998;124:301–303.
21. Cernea CR, Ferraz AR, Nishio S, Dutra A Jr, Hojaij FC, dos Santos LR. Surgical anatomy of the external branch of the superior laryngeal nerve. *Head Neck.* 1992;14:380–383.
22. Raffaelli M, Iacobone M, Henry JF. The "false" nonrecurrent inferior laryngeal nerve. *Surgery.* 2000;128:1082–1087.
23. Kiray A, Arman C, Naderi S, Guvencer M, Korman E. Surgical anatomy of the cervical sympathetic trunk. *Clin Anat.* 2005;18:179–185.
24. Sim E, Vaccaro AR, Berzlanovich A, Thaler H, Ullrich CG. Fenestration of the extracranial vertebral artery: review of the literature. *Spine.* 2001;26:E139–E142.
25. Hong JT, Park DK, Lee MJ, Kim SW, An HS. Anatomical variations of the vertebral artery segment in the lower cervical spine: analysis by three-dimensional computed tomography angiography. *Spine.* 2008;33:2422–2426.
26. Vaswani M, Waldron HA. The earliest case of extracranial aneurysm of the vertebral artery. *Br J Neurosurg.* 1997;11:164–165.
27. Bruneau M, Cornelius JF, Marneffe V, Triffaux M, George B. Anatomical variations of the v2 segment of the vertebral artery. *Neurosurgery.* 2006;59:ONS20-24; discussion ONS20-24.
28. Tokuda K, Miyasaka K, Abe H, Abe S, Takei H, Sugimoto S, Tsuru M. Anomalous atlantoaxial portions of vertebral and posterior inferior cerebellar arteries. *Neuroradiology.* 1985;27:410–413.
29. Cagnie B, Barbaix E, Vinck E, D'Herde K, Cambier D. Extrinsic risk factors for compromised blood flow in the vertebral artery: anatomical observations of the transverse foramina from C3 to C7. *Surg Radiol Anat.* 2005;27:312–316.
30. Tubbs RS, Loukas M, Remy AC, Shoja MM, Salter EG, Oakes WJ. The vertebral nerve revisited. *Clin Anat.* 2007;20:644–647.
31. Weintraub MI, Khoury A. Critical neck position as an independent risk factor for posterior circulation stroke. A magnetic resonance angiographic analysis. *J Neuroimaging* 1995;5:16–22.

32. Pamphlett R, Raisanen J, Kum-Jew S. Vertebral artery compression resulting from head movement: a possible cause of the sudden infant death syndrome. *Pediatrics.* 1999;103:460–468.
33. Hong JM, Chung CS, Bang OY, Yong SW, Joo IS, Huh K. Vertebral artery dominance contributes to basilar artery curvature and peri-vertebrobasilar junctional infarcts. *J Neurol Neurosurg Psychiatry.* 2009;80:1087–1092.
34. Smith AS, Bellon JR. Parallel and spiral flow patterns of vertebral artery contributions to the basilar artery. *Am J Neuroradiol.* 1995;16:1587–1591.
35. Wilkinson IM. The vertebral artery. Extracranial and intracranial structure. *Arch Neurol.* 1972;27:392–396.
36. Peltier J, Toussaint P, Deramond H, et al. The dural crossing of the vertebral artery. *Surg Radiol Anat SRA.* 2003;25:305–310.
37. Krabbe-Hartkamp MJ, van der Grond J, de Leeuw FE, et al. Circle of Willis: morphologic variation on three-dimensional time-of-flight MR angiograms. *Radiology.* 1998;207:103–111.
38. Yilmaz E, Ilgit E, Taner D. Primitive persistent carotid-basilar and carotid-vertebral anastomoses: a report of seven cases and a review of the literature. *Clin Anat.* 1995;8:36–43.
39. Anderson RA, Sondheimer FK. Rare carotid-vertebrobasilar anastomoses with notes on the differentiation between proatlantal and hypoglossal arteries. *Neuroradiology.* 1976;11:113–118.

CHAPTER 2

Differences between the Carotid and Vertebral Systems

For the vascular surgeon, the differences between the carotid and vertebral systems are more relevant than their similarities. Both arteries supply the brain, they run roughly parallel courses in the neck, and, once they enter the cranium, they lose much of their elastic components and their walls become thin and frail. The similarities end there.

The typical lesion of the ICA, the atheromatous plaque in the bulb, is localized there because of the peculiar geometry of the bifurcation. A specific lesion of the VA, compression/occlusion with head rotation, is the consequence of its course inside a mobile musculoskeletal tunnel in the neck.

DIVERGENCE VS. CONVERGENCE

The layouts of the carotid and vertebral systems are opposite. The CCA and the ICA bifurcate. The VA, on the contrary, converges with the other VA to become a single BA.[i] The fact that both VAs supply the BA presents a problem when we are trying to determine which VA is the *source of an embolic infarction* in the cerebellum or brain stem because an embolus lodging in the BA or any of its branches could have originated from either VA. An exception to this statement exists in those individuals who have one hypoplastic VA (missing part of its fourth segment). The embolus in the latter case would have had to travel through the opposite, normal VA.

The ICA and the VA *occlude* with different patterns. The ICA usually occludes its full length from its origin to the siphon because it has no significant branches between these two points. The VA tends to occlude in a segmental manner involving part or most of its cervical portion, but then, it reconstitutes at the level of C2–C1 by collaterals supplied by the occipital or cervical ascending arteries. This allows us to reconstruct an occluded VA at this distal level, something we cannot do for the ICA.

DIFFERENT PATHOLOGY

Our *understanding* of the carotid and vertebral systems is dissimilar. The protagonism that each system has in the development of a stroke was proven for the carotid territory

---

[i] There are other arterial convergence arrangements in the cerebrospinal arterial supply. The anterior spinal artery, the first branch of the VA after it becomes intradural, joins with its opposite to form the single anterior spinal artery. The anterior and posterior communicating arteries merge flow from both ICAs and the BA.

in 1951 by Fisher[1,2] and for the vertebral territory in 1956 by Hutchinson and Yates.[3] Both studies showed that embolization could occur from plaques that had degenerative features such as ulceration, intraplaque hemorrhage, or superimposed thrombus. It has always been possible to inspect directly the carotid lesions in the operating room and at autopsy and this has allowed the correlation of specific features of the carotid plaque, such as hemorrhage, surface thrombus, and ulceration, with the incidence of clinical symptoms. In the VA, on the contrary, because the operations we do are transpositions or bypasses, neither surgeons nor pathologists have a chance to study the offending specimen.

The *mechanism of brain infarction* in the carotid and vertebral territories is either low flow or embolism. In the ICA territory, at least 75% of strokes or transient ischemic attacks (TIAs) are secondary to embolism from a plaque. In the VA territory, 70% of the ischemic symptoms are caused by low flow and only 30% are embolic. The reason for this disparity is the high incidence of flow-arresting extrinsic compression found in patients that experience vertebral basilar ischemia (VBI) from head and neck movements. This bone-compressive pathology that results in low-flow VBI is not seen in the carotid arteries.

An enduring flaw in the general understanding of VB pathology is to attribute its clinical manifestations solely to low flow and to not include microembolization as a common cause of TIA or stroke in the VB territory. There is also a clinical concept often invoked in the VB territory that lacks a pathological correlate: that of "watershed infarction." The implication of this term is that this territory by being the boundary of perfusion between the carotid and basilar flow is more susceptible to low-flow infarction. The term "watershed" may be appealing as a metaphor but it does not describe a "parting of the waters": it just designates a boundary where the anterior and the posterior perfusion encounter each other. By now we know, and we see it in angiograms, that this boundary is not fixed and moves forward and backward depending on the relative perfusion pressure of the ICA and BA. More to the point, the detailed autopsy series of Castaigne,[4] Amarenco,[5] and Pessin[6] proved that *most infarcts in the VB territory are embolic* and, less frequently, may be caused by thrombus growing on a preexisting plaque located in an intracranial artery. Neuropathologists have not found infarctions along the presumed watershed boundary, without identifying a causative embolus or thrombus attached to an intracranial arterial lesion. It is reasonable to conclude that low-flow "watershed infarction" between the anterior and posterior territories does not exist.

The *outcome of infarctions* in the carotid territory is different from that in the VB system: death from posterior infarctions is three times higher than that from anterior ones.

Imaging of the carotid lesion has been possible since Egas Moniz did the first cerebral angiogram in 1927. Currently, duplex scanning, CTA, and MRA are the standard methods for imaging the carotid bifurcation. For carotid lesions outside the field of view of the ultrasound (US) equipment, we have CTAs that produce detailed images that can be studied in three dimensions. In the VA territory, duplex ultrasound studies give us only information regarding the presence of a functioning VA and the direction of flow through it. Proximal VA lesions may not be seen in conventional four-vessel arteriograms unless an exaggerated oblique projection is used. For the diagnosis of dynamic compression of the VA, a special angiogram is needed that requires positioning of the head in symptom-triggering position (see Section "Dynamic Compression of the Vertebral Artery (Bow Hunter Syndrome)" in Chapter 3). CTA provides a good outline of VA lesions and of their relationship to neighboring vertebral bone.

We have had CTs to visualize infarctions in the carotid territory for more than 30 years. Medullary and brain stem infarcts are generally too small and surrounded by dense bone to be seen in CTs. In order to see the small infarcts in the posterior circulation resulting from VA microembolization, we had to wait for MR to be available in the 1980s. Only then, the possibility that infarction could be due to microemboli could be entertained.

UNEQUAL CLINICAL COURSE

The carotid-supplied hemispheres express symptoms of ischemia with a precise unilateral topography, the vertebrobasilar-supplied posterior brain displays alternating symptoms of diffuse representation.

The term "insufficiency" is generally used when describing ischemic symptoms arising from the posterior fossa. "Insufficiency" implies a paucity of flow, a flow rate that is inadequate to the demands of the territory being supplied. Because it applies to only one of the mechanisms of ischemia, it prompts the clinician to look for a flow-limiting lesion rather than a potential source for microemboli. It is desirable to abandon the term "insufficiency" that, in view of what we know today, is stale and inadequate. It should be replaced by the noun "ischemia," as was done a quarter of a century ago when describing carotid or coronary symptoms.

Finally, surgical access to the CA and that to the VA are different. The CA, traveling under skin and muscle in the neck, has easy access for surgical treatment. This is not the situation in the VA where surgical accessibility in the low neck is more demanding than in the carotid case, a difficulty that increases when the artery is exposed higher, at skull base level.

REFERENCES

1. Fisher M. Occlusion of the internal carotid artery. *Arch Neurol Psychiatry.* 1951;65:346–377.
2. Fisher M. Occlusion of the carotid artery. *Arch Neurol Psychiatry.* 1954;72:187–204.
3. Hutchinson EC, Yates PO. The cervical portion of the vertebral artery: a clinico-pathological study. *Brain.* 1956;79:319–331.
4. Castaigne P, Lhermitte F, Gautier JC, et al. Arterial occlusions in the vertebro-basilar system. A study of 44 patients with post-mortem data. *Brain.* 1973;96:133–154.
5. Amarenco P, Hauw JJ. Cerebellar infarction in the territory of the anterior and inferior cerebellar artery. A clinicopathological study of 20 cases. *Neurology.* 1990;40:1383–1390.
6. Pessin MS. Posterior cerebral-artery disease and occipital ischemia. In *Vertebrobasilar Aretrial Disease.* Eds. R. Berguer and L. Caplan. Quality Medical Publishing, St. Louis 1991. pp. 66–75.

CHAPTER 3

The Pathology

LESION

Duplex Ultrasonography (US) is currently the standard tool for the initial evaluation of a patient suspected of having carotid artery disease. The rating of carotid artery disease by US is based upon recorded velocity waveforms and B-mode images. The latter are generally enhanced with color flow coding.

There are some instances where US does not provide a full assessment of the condition of the patient; the most frequent being (1) carotid lesions located outside the space limited by the jaw above and the clavicle below. Changes in waveform and velocity recorded at the bifurcation can detect the existence of these lesions within the chest or cranium, but they cannot define their significance; (2) a heavily calcified bifurcation that does not permit reliable US imaging or velocity sampling; (3) fibromuscular dysplasia (FMD) or dissection of the ICA that tends to occur distal to the area that can be interrogated by US.

CTA is the diagnostic tool most often used to settle questions that cannot be clarified by US. It is less expensive than MRA and is available at most institutions. A CTA of the head and neck gives information regarding the extra- and intracranial course of both ICA and VA as well as pertinent details regarding the completeness or otherwise of the circle of Willis. The accompanying CT provides a useful scan of the brain parenchyma.

Today non-contrast CT and CTA are the most useful tools in planning an operation or an intervention in the carotid or vertebral arteries of a symptomatic patient, excepting patients with VBI secondary to neck rotation (see below). Modern multisection CT machines can produce a CTA, including post-processing manipulations, in 30 minutes.[1] The efficiency of these new systems is quite relevant to the initiation of treatment after acute stroke because most protocols require not exceeding a 3-hour window from the appearance of symptoms before establishing therapy.

The incidence of *silent infarction* in asymptomatic patients with carotid bifurcation disease is 17%.[2] If, in addition to having a known carotid plaque, a patient has experienced a TIA, there is a 45% probability of finding an infarction on CT.[3] This high probability of unsuspected infarction should have made it mandatory to obtain a non-contrast CT before recruiting a patient to any randomized study that attempts to compare the efficiency or risk of a carotid procedure. The absence of a baseline CT marrs the interpretation of many randomized studies since we could never know if the lesions that were observed in follow-up were present at the time of recruitment.

Although we think of a TIA as a temporary and reversible perfusion defect, up to *34% of patients who have TIAs actually have an appropriate infarct*[3] seen in CT.

A CTA obtained prior to a CEA in a symptomatic patient will allow us to rule out lesions (in the common carotid artery or carotid syphon), which are outside the field surveyed by the US. A CTA will also show the location and size of the infarctions that we can anticipate finding in one-third of the patients with clinical TIAs.

MRA has been proposed as the diagnostic tool to use when calcium deposits block the US. But MRA is not ubiquitous and is expensive. Furthermore, it tends to overestimate the severity of lesions[4] located in a segment where flow abruptly changes direction, as in the origin of the ICA.

Angiography is seldom used nowadays in the workup of ICA atherosclerotic disease but it may still be needed to evaluate plaques in the intracranial segment or in the supraortic trunks (SAT). Arteriography may be necessary for the evaluation of some aneurysms and AV fistulae.

The usefulness of CTA is limited in the workup of patients with VBI. If a patient has had a TIA or a stroke of VB distribution, the CT may show a cerebellar infarction but it is unlikely to show the minute pontine infarcts that follow the occlusion of the thin perforating arteries supplying the pons. The dense bone that surrounds the brain stem causes refraction artifacts that dampen the optical resolution of the CT in this area. CTA studies with rotation/extension of the head are not feasible because it is difficult to access the patient's head and neck and to maintain the head in the trigger position while scanning. MRA, on the other hand, is the best imaging technique to assess the parenchyma of the VB territory particularly to detect the small infarcts that develop in the brain stem that is supplied by small perforating arteries. Patients with VBI triggered by head and neck rotation need to be evaluated by dynamic arteriography, as described in Section "Dynamic Compression of the Vertebral Artery (Bow Hunter Syndrome) p.57."

COMPOSITION OF THE PLAQUE

The classic and now outdated ACAS and NASCET studies rated the severity of a plaque on the basis of percent diameter stenosis (although the referential diameter to which the narrowed lumen was compared was different for each of these studies) and showed a correlation between the severity of the stenosis and the likelihood of brain ischemia. Percent diameter reduction is of standard and general use in describing the severity of an occlusive lesion: it is a metric easy to define and can be used to describe the size of a plaque with any of the current imaging tools: US, CTA, MRA, and angiography. Bur percent stenosis describes only the relative size of the plaque in reference to the lumen of the artery. There is no linearity between the size of the plaque and its virulence.

From NASCET arose the recommendation to restrict surgery to symptomatic plaques rated at greater than 75% diameter stenosis. While this heuristic has become accepted medical practice, there are other characteristics of the plaque, more relevant than the percent diameter stenoses, that have been left out of the decision tree. This fixation on the percent stenosis as the single indicator of the severity of a carotid plaque in most randomized studies has translated into a lack of appreciation of the role played by other equally relevant factors, such as the presence of hypoechoic areas and intraplaque hemorrhage, the rupture of the fibrous cap, or the presence of ulceration.

The largest mechanical stresses bearing on the plaque occur in its fibrous cap. These stresses increase when the lipid core is near the fibrous cap and may cause the cap to rupture, embolize, and result in brain ischemia. If, in addition, there are areas of discrete calcification, the peak stresses may increase by as much as 70%.[5]

The work of Russell,[6] Biasi,[7] Sabetai[8] and others showed the clinical relevance of assessing the ultrasonic density of plaque by gray scale median (GSM) rating. The ICAROS study,[7] done in patients undergoing angioplasty and stenting of the ICA, adopted an arbitrary value of 25 GSM as the boundary between hyperechoic and hypoechoic plaques. Plaques with a low GSM value have a high lipid and hemorrhagic content and are more likely to result in a stroke (microembolization) following angioplasty and stenting.

The characteristics that contribute to the morbidity of a plaque can be summarized as follows: little fibrous tissue, large areas of lipid content or presence of intraplaque hemorrhage, and rupture of the cap with resulting ulceration.

Nearly all ischemic events caused by a plaque result from particulate embolization of the contents of an ulcer or from the detachment of platelet clusters or thrombus that have formed in the downstream boundary of a plaque. Only a minority of ischemic events are caused by the restriction of flow imposed by the plaque. Given that older plaques are larger and contain more degenerative features, it is not surprising that there is some correlation between plaque size and plaque morbidity. But size alone should not be the only criterion to gauge the potential threat of a plaque. A symptomatic patient with a carotid US showing morbid features (ulceration, intraplaque hemorrhage, etc.) in the appropriate carotid should be considered for operation/intervention regardless of whether it satisfies the 70% to 99% criterion. On the other hand, there is no evidence that a 75% stenosis caused by a mostly fibrous lesion (intimal hyperplasia) in an asymptomatic patient requires an endarterectomy to improve the chances that the patient will live stroke-free for the remainder of his life.

FIBROMUSCULAR DYSPLASIA

FMD is a disease of medium-sized muscular arteries affecting their middle and distal segments; their proximal segment is generally spared. FMD is most commonly found in the renal arteries and is followed in frequency by the ICA and VA. It affects predominantly young and middle-aged women. Genetic and familial studies[9] suggest that FMD is transmitted as an autosomal dominant trait with reduced penetrance in males. Most patients with FMD of the VA also have FMD lesions in their ICA. If a patient presents with FMD of an ICA, the chance that the contralateral ICA will be affected is approximately 50%. FMD of the ICA is far more common among relatives of patients who have renal FMD. Patients with FMD of the carotid and vertebral arteries also have a high incidence (20% to 50%) of "berry" type intracranial ICA aneurysms.[10]

The ICA and the VA usually display the characteristic changes of FMD at about the level of C2 and this high location makes US inadequate to visualize the lesion. In older reports, angiography was the diagnostic tool commonly used. In modern series, the diagnosis of FMD is made by MRA or CTA.

Three types of FMD are classically described.[11] Most of the cases fall under the medial or perimedial FMD that causes the iconic "string of beads" appearance. The ridges are made of fibroproliferative tissue and the outpouchings (microaneurysms) occur where smooth muscle is deficient or where the internal elastic membrane is missing. Intimal FMD, which results in focal concentric stenosis, occurs in less than 10% of cases. Adventitial hyperplasia is the rarest form.

CAROTID AND VERTEBRAL ARTERY DISSECTION

Although we talk about an "intimal flap" in dissections of the ICA or VA, the plane of dissection is not beneath the intima but rather within the media. In the extracranial ICA and VA (muscular arteries), the flap (inner layer) is made up of intima, internal elastic membrane, and a thin layer of media. The remaining wall (outer layer) is composed of the remaining media and adventitia.

A dissection is typically described as a progressing intramural hematoma resulting from a rent of the inner layer of the artery through which blood insinuates itself into the media. And indeed, all recent dissections have blood within the media, but, in some cases, the intimal tear that is presumed to be the source of this medial hematoma is not found. It is believed that these latter patients may have experienced shear forces in the media that tore the radially laid vasa vasora causing the intramural hemorrhage. In most cases, the dissecting hematoma will develop a distal tear through which the hematoma decompresses into the arterial blood stream. Thrombus within the false lumen may embolize downstream through this distal tear.

In the ICA and VA, the plane of dissection is beneath the internal elastic membrane and therefore the flap is thin (Fig. 3.1). The intramural hematoma makes the thin flap bulge into the lumen causing the latter to narrow ("string sign" in arteriograms) or to occlude. This intramural hematoma may continue to grow, distending the cleavage layer it occupies and eventually expanding under the adventitia. This sequence of events usually results in an aneurysm.[12] If the hematoma ruptures through the adventitia, a false aneurysm will develop.

Dissections of the IA or CCA are either due to trauma (Figs. 3.2 and 3.3) or due to the extension of a Type A aortic dissection.

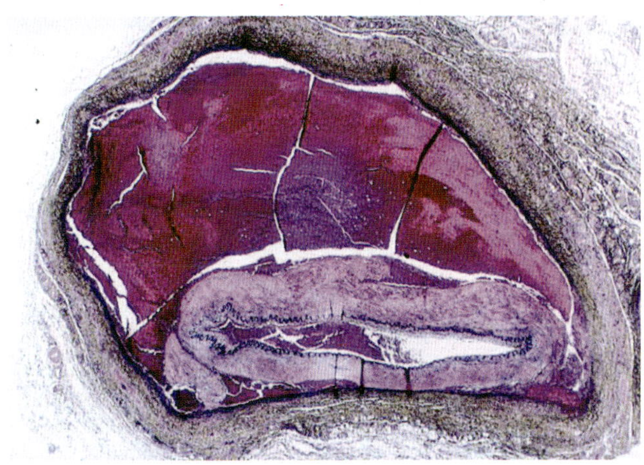

FIGURE 3.1. Cross-section of a dissection in the cervical ICA.

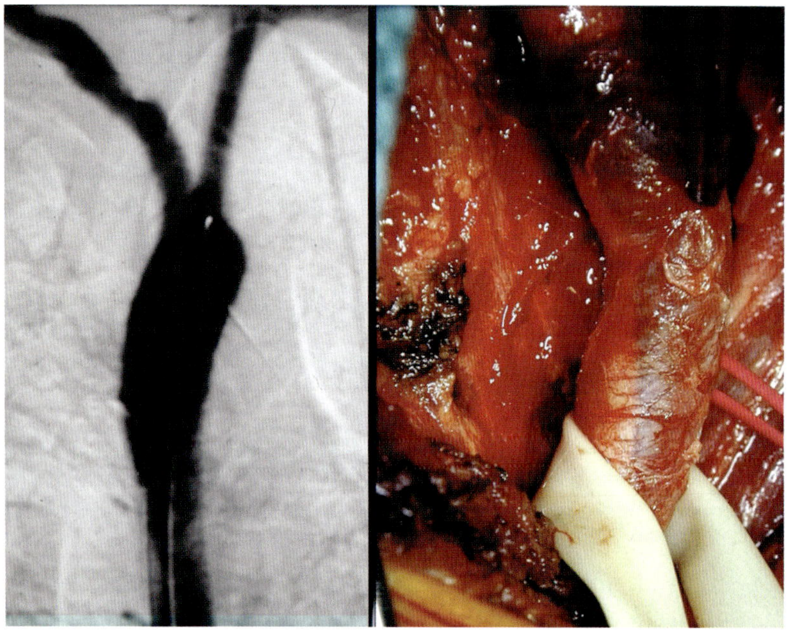

FIGURE 3.2. Traumatic dissection (car crash) of the IA and CCA. The operative photograph shows the dissecting hematoma in the IA.

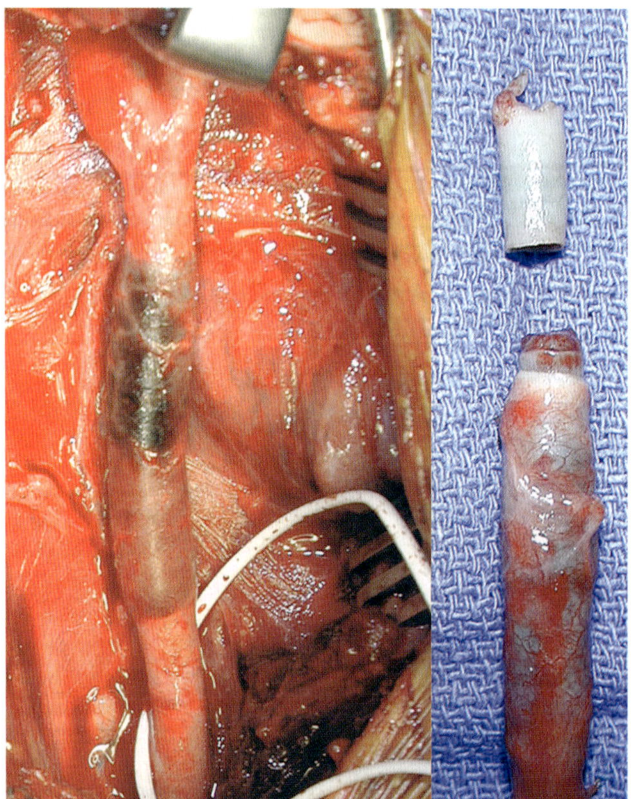

FIGURE 3.3. Traumatic dissection of the CCA (compression by a mechanical elevator platform). The dissected cylinder core (top right) embolized the ICA.

In their *intracranial* segments, the ICA and the VA have a much thinner wall and, as a consequence, the dissecting hematoma may rupture through the adventitia resulting in a subarachnoid hemorrhage, most often fatal.[13] Dissection of the intracranial ICA or VA is rare but carries a grim prognosis. Intracranial dissection if the ICA is rare in adults but more common in children.[14] For reasons unknown, boys experience 73% of all the dissection seen in children and this male predominance is found in dissections that are preceded by trauma (14%) and in those that are "spontaneous" (86%).

The considerations that follow apply to the far more common *extracranial dissections* of the ICA and VA. There must be either a new applied mechanical force or a tissue defect from an underlying arteriopathy to explain a dissection of the ICA. This latter proposition is supported by the fact that in spontaneous ICA dissection we find a synchronous dissection of the other ICA or of the VA in 6% to 15% of the cases. Presumably in these latter cases the ICAs and VAs would share the arteriopathy that eventually resulted in the symptomatic dissection of the one ICA. Furthermore, the ICAs of patients with spontaneous dissection display a higher than normal Young's elastic modulus and circumferential wall stress in both the dissected and non-dissected sides.

However, patients with spontaneous carotid dissection have normal elastic parameters in their aorta and radial arteries.[15] Ehler-Danlos patients,[16] who are at increased risk for dissection or rupture of their vascular lesions, have a thinner intima-media layer and higher circumferential wall stress in their carotid arteries but, again, the elastic parameters of their radial arteries are normal. These findings suggest that the matrix defect in these cases is confined to the arteries supplying the brain.

There is a statistically weak association between spontaneous dissection of the ICA and connective tissue disorders such as aortic root dilatation, intracranial aneurysm, and FMD.[17,18] Lesions of FMD are seen in 15% of patients with spontaneous ICA dissection and 5% of patients with spontaneous ICA dissection have a family member with a history of dissection of the aorta or its branches. A hypothesis proposed for this association, weak as it is, is that the latter arteries share some unknown matrix defect with the ICA.

A load straining the wall of the carotid artery results first in the failure of the intima-media layer. Such failure may be caused by a "normal" load on a weakened wall (spontaneous) (Fig. 3.4) or a very high load on a normal arterial wall (trauma) (Fig. 3.5). The sequence of failure of the two layers can be shown (Fig. 3.6) by placing a strip of CCA in a tensile strength machine and progressively straining it.[19] The first layer to tear is the intima-media layer. As straining continues, additional tears develop in this layer and, eventually, the adventitia-media layer ruptures.

The dissection of the ICA generally stops at the entrance of the bony temporal canal where the adventitia of the carotid is bound to the surrounding periosteum (Fig. 3.7). Rarely, an ICA dissection results in multiple aneurysms (Fig. 3.8). Similarly, the dissection of the extracranial VA usually stops at the point where the artery penetrates the duramater and exchanges collagen anchors with it. In 10% of cases a dissection of either ICA or VA may extend intracranially. The distal extension of an intracranial VA dissection is extremely risky: if it reaches the BA the mortality is 90%.[20]

ICA/VA dissection is the cause of 20% of the strokes seen in people younger than 50 years old.[12] By far the most common dissection site is the high cervical

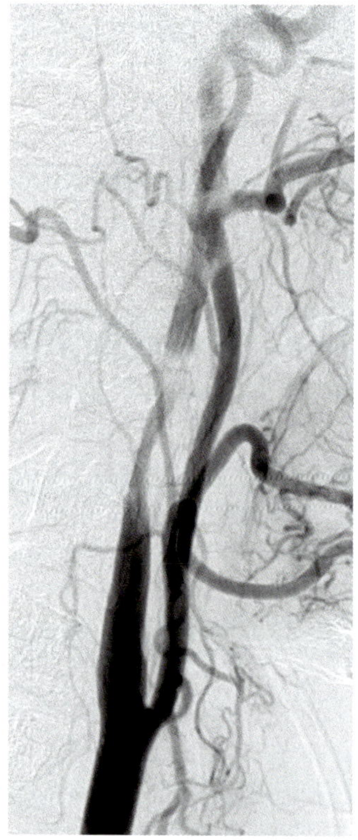

FIGURE 3.4. Spontaneous dissection of the ICA at C2.

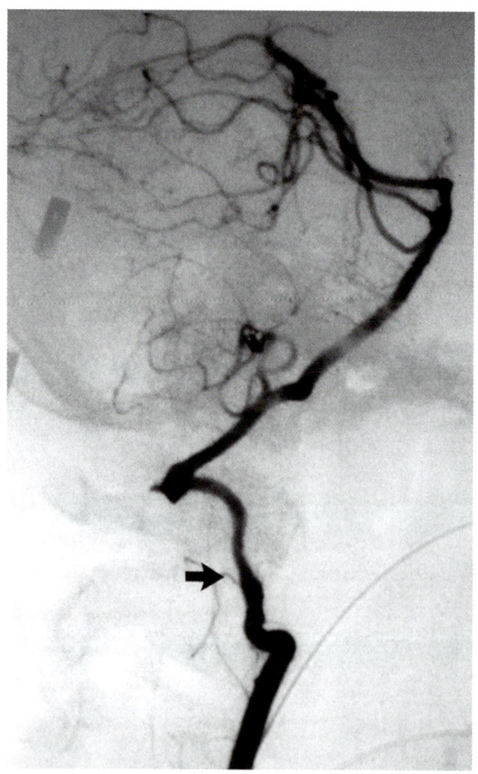

FIGURE 3.5. Traumatic dissection of the V3 segment (arrow) noted in a young athlete after chiropractic manipulation. Note the ventriculostomy tube already in place. Patient died 12 hours after admission.

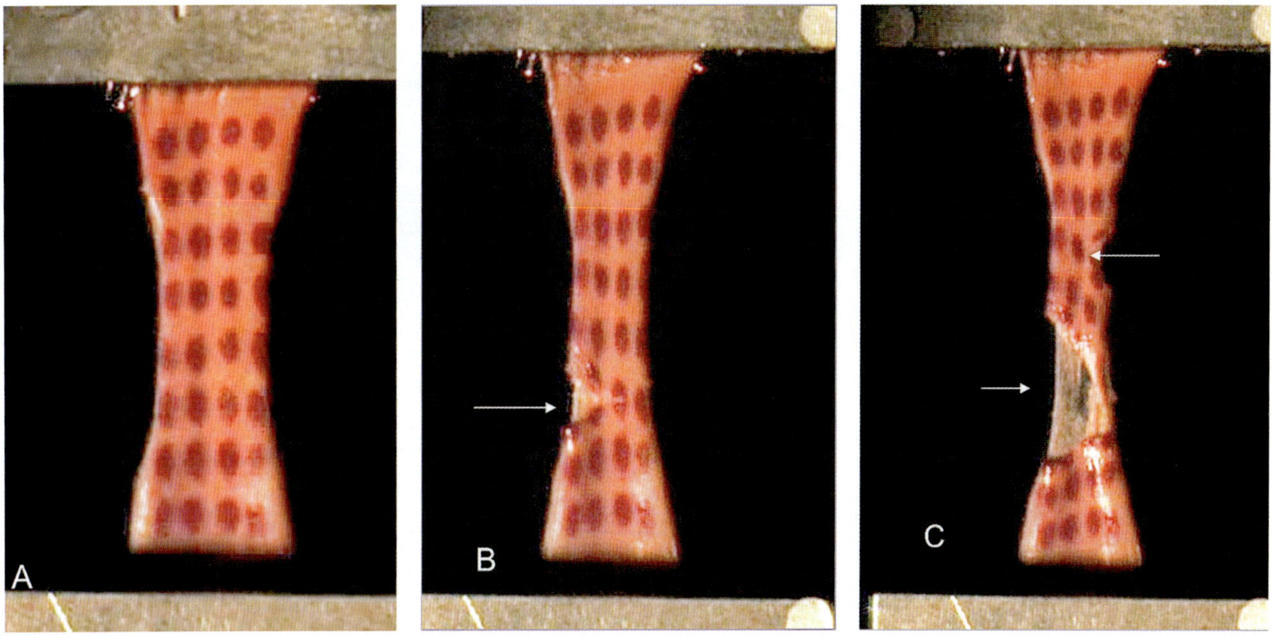

FIGURE 3.6. A strip of ICA (with location dots placed on the intima) is stretched between the jaws of a tensile strength machine (**A**). Note the initial fractures (**B**, **C**) of the inner layers (arrows) that preceded the rupture of the specimen. (Reproduced with permission from Stemper BD, Yoganandan N, Pintar FA. Methodology to study intimal failure mechanics in human internal carotid arteries. *J Biomech*. 2005;38:2491–2496.)

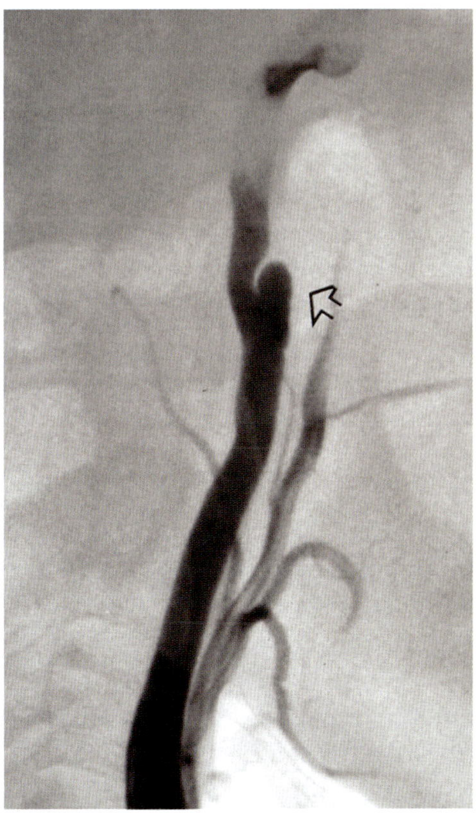

FIGURE 3.7. The dissecting hematoma in the ICA stops at the carotid canal (arrow).

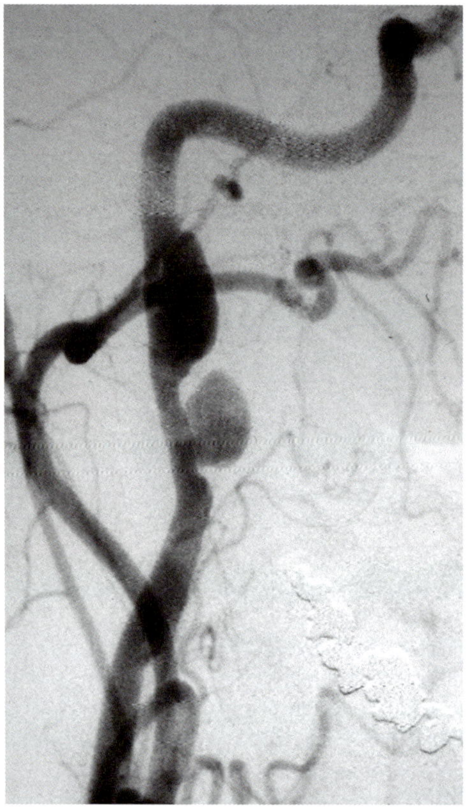

FIGURE 3.8. Unusual development of two sequential aneurysms from an ICA dissection.

portion of the ICA/VA. In the ICA this preferred location is the consequence of its close relationship with the transverse process of C1 (Fig. 3.4). For the VA it is the result of the exceptional mobility of the C1–C2 joint that can mechanically stress the artery (Fig. 3.5). Of these extracranial dissections, one-third of them follow blunt trauma but in two-thirds of cases we call them "spontaneous" because no proximate cause is associated with their appearance.

Most imaging studies done in patients with ICA dissection in the last 20 years have used MR.[21] But a comparative study[22] of different modalities concluded that CTA offers the better spatial resolution for the local features of ICA dissection (seeing the flap, identifying the thrombus in the false lumen, etc). MR, on the other hand, is better at assessing the embolic consequences of dissection (infarction) in the brain parenchyma.

The typical *presentation of an ICA dissection* is head and neck pain and a partial (miosis and ptosis) Horner's.[23,i] Patients with *VA dissection* present with pain in the occipital and posterior neck regions that may be misinterpreted as being of musculoskeletal origin.

A few days later (on an average four) brain ischemic symptoms appear, most commonly a stroke (84%) and less frequently a TIA. In both ICA and VA dissection, there is an interval of several days between the appearance of local symptoms (neck pain,

---

[i] Facial anhydrosis is not present because the sympathetic innervations of the sweat glands of the face surround the ECA that is not involved in the dissection.

Horner's) and the development of brain ischemic symptoms. This delay is the time it takes for the dissecting hematoma to occlude the lumen or to release thromboembolic fragments from the initial tear or progress distally and, through a distal tear, reenter the true lumen discharging fragments of thrombus into it. The end-organ effects in ICA dissection are hemispheric or retinal ischemia. In VA dissection, the infarction will be in the brain stem (lateral medullary syndrome), thalamus, cerebellum, and occipital lobes.

One-half of patients with spontaneous ICA dissection develop a brain infarction and this infarct is embolic in 90% of cases[ii]; not due to low flow as it is often surmised.[24,25]

The rate of clinical redissection of the same ICA or VA is reported to be low from 0.4%[26] to 8.0%.[27] Redissection is more common in patients with underlying arteriopathy.[28] It is believed that an ICA/VA that has dissected and eventually healed has added enough scarring to its media to prevent the reoccurrence of separation of the wall layers. This incidence of redissection turns out to be higher when the patients who have had a dissection are followed with routine imaging. In this latter group, 6% will have a silent synchronous dissection of the opposite ICA or VA and 25% will eventually show a redissection or a new dissection in an ICA or VA.

Most ICA/VA dissections will recanalize, or "remodel," in 6 months regardless of whether the dissection had resulted in a double channel, a stenosis, or an occlusion. About one-third of the false aneurysms are seen to decrease in size with time. Recanalization of a VA dissection is seen in 60% of patients within 6 months.

Treatment of Spontaneous Dissection of the Internal Carotid and Vertebral Arteries

The consensual treatment of spontaneous dissection is anticoagulant therapy, although the superiority of anticoagulant versus antiplatelet therapy has not been proven.[29] Because recanalization and remodeling takes place 3 to 6 months after the appearance of symptoms, anticoagulant therapy is generally maintained during this interval. The use of anticoagulants is questioned in VA dissection, most particularly in those patients in whom the dissection has extended intracranially, because of the threat of potentially lethal subarachnoid hemorrhage. Experience with thrombolysis is controversial.

If anticoagulant/antiplatelet therapy does not control an unstable dissection and the patient continues to suffer embolization from it, intervention should be considered either by means of a bypass or a stent (Figs. 3.9 and 3.10). The false aneurysm that may follow an ICA dissection may continue to expand or may be the source of emboli. In this case, it will require intervention either with a stent or with a bypass.

In summary, patients with spontaneous ICA/VA dissection have abnormal elastic parameters in their dissected and non-dissected craniocervical arteries. The downstream effects of a dissection, usually brain infarction, are embolic and not due to low flow. Extracranial dissection of the ICA or VA is empirically managed with anticoagulants or antiplatelet agents.

[ii] Transcranial Doppler shows microembolic "hits" in the MCA in 60% of patients with ICA dissection.

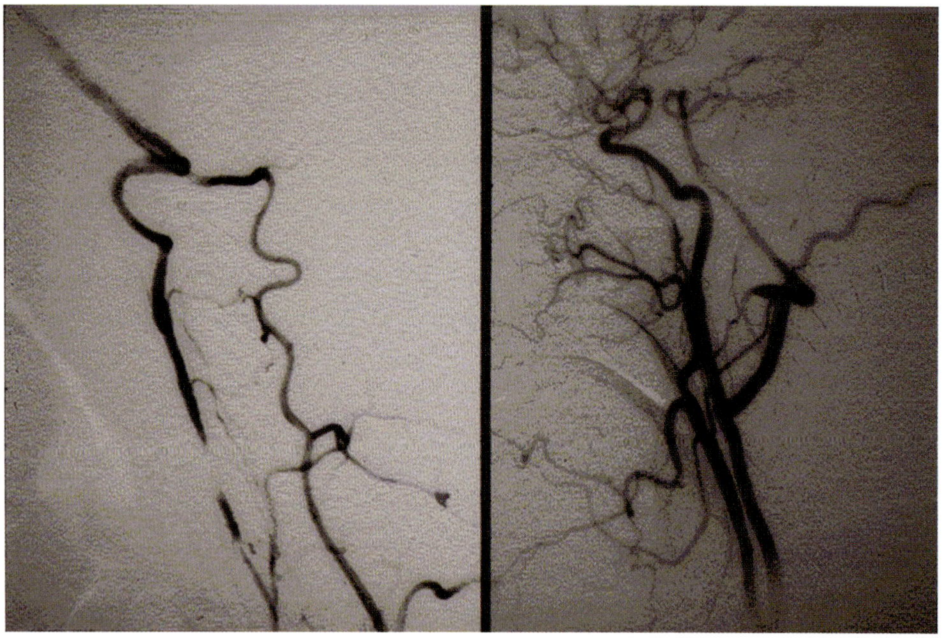

FIGURE 3.9. A dissected VA (left) that continued to embolize in spite of appropriate full anticoagulation was treated with exclusion of the dissected segment by a vein bypass from the ICA to the suboccipital (C0–C1) VA segment (right).

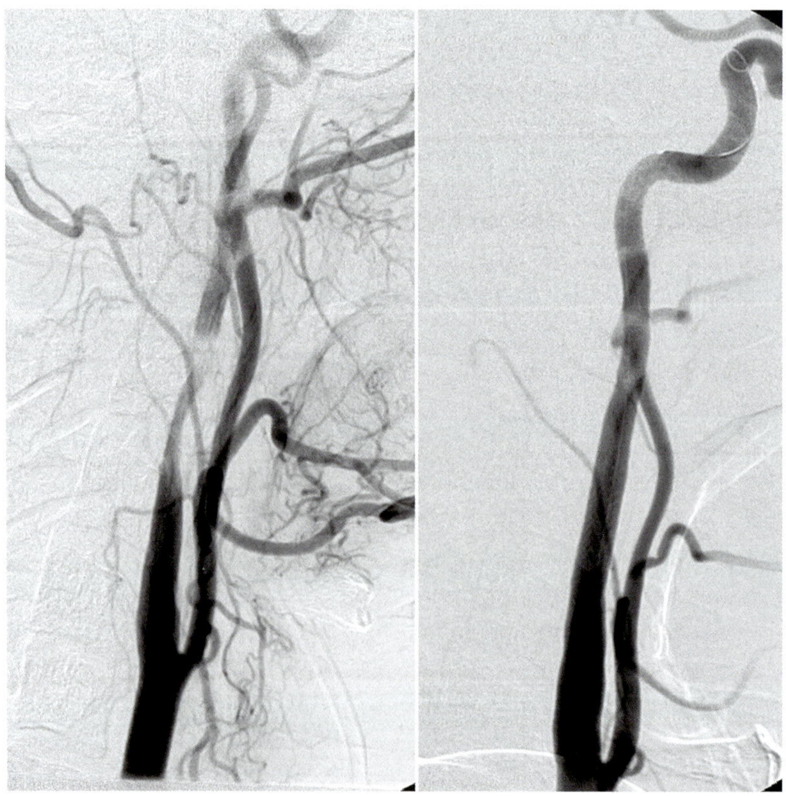

FIGURE 3.10. This young woman had occluded the opposite carotid following an episode of spontaneous dissection. She presented 1 year later with a new dissection in her only patent ICA. She was treated with a stent (right).

ATHEROSCLEROTIC AND DYSPLASTIC CAROTID AND VERTEBRAL ANEURYSMS

With syphilis gone from aortic pathology, aneurysms of the IA nowadays are either a consequence of trauma or part of a connective tissue disorder that involves also the arch of the aorta. Post-traumatic aneurysms are generally the result of car accidents with the steering wheel impacting on the sternum causing blunt injury to the IA (Fig. 3.11).

The finding of an IA aneurysm without a history of trauma should alert the surgeon to the high probability that the dilated IA is likely to be part of more generalized aortic arch disease. Any attempt to treat such a patient with an exclusion bypass based on the ascending aorta is bound to cause a dissection of the aortic arch, a situation that is unmanageable in a patient who is not under cardiopulmonary bypass.[iii]

Carotid aneurysmectomy represents only 0.1% to 2.2% of all carotid procedures and carotid aneurysms are only 0.2% to 1% of all arterial aneurysms.[30] There have been differing opinions as to what constitutes an aneurysm at this level, given the natural enlargement of the artery at the bulb. De Jong[31] has proposed that an enlarged

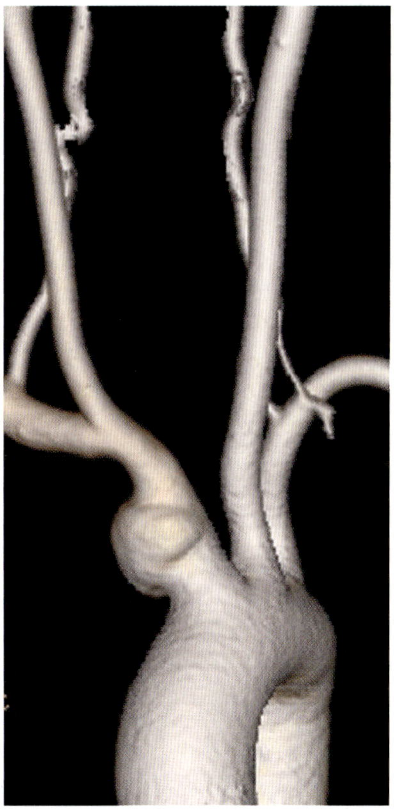

FIGURE 3.11. A head-on collision caused this IA aneurysm diagnosed 2 years after the accident. It was treated with a bypass from ascending aorta to IA.

[iii] Figure 3.12 shows the CTA of a 70-year-old woman who presented with signs of tracheal compression by what I thought was a primary aneurysm of the IA. When the exclusion clamp was placed on the ascending aorta to construct the proximal anastomosis of an exclusion bypass, a large retrograde dissection involving both coronaries ensued. Although the patient was placed immediately on cardiopulmonary bypass she did not survive the massive myocardial ischemia.

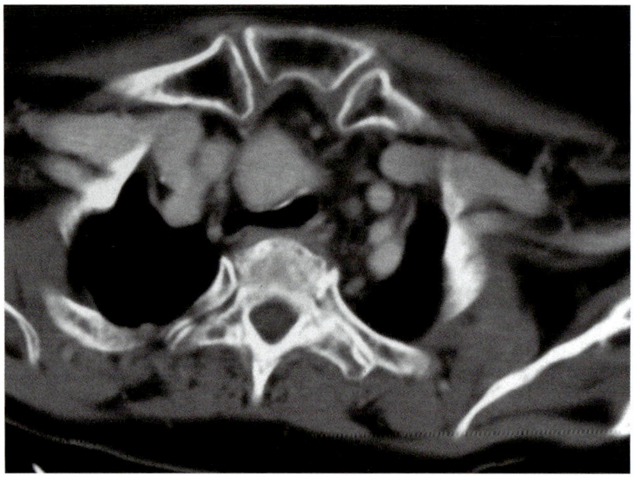

FIGURE 3.12. Tracheal compression by an aneurysmal IA.

bulb is to be called an aneurysm if it has a >200% diameter than that of the more distal ICA, or if it is >150% than that of the distal CCA.

Carotid aneurysm series in the literature describe different types of aneurysmal disease. In older reports, the majority of carotid aneurysms were either mycotic or traumatic. In series from medical centers with a busy trauma unit, most carotid aneurysms are false aneurysms following trauma. Atherosclerotic aneurysms of the ICA are rare. The large series of McCollum[32] (USA) describes a 44% incidence of atherosclerotic aneurysm, but no instance of dysplastic aneurysm. A series by El-Sabrout (USA)[33] mentions two possible dysplasias among 67 aneurysms of other etiology. In contraposition, the European series of Moreau,[34] Rosset,[35] and Faggioli[30] list dysplastic aneurysms as their most frequent group.

A *dysplastic aneurysm* is typically located in the mid or high cervical ICA; it is saccular in shape (Fig. 3.13) and often associated with elongation and loops of the remaining extracranial ICA. Their lining is often normal in areas not covered by thrombus which is found in about half of them (Fig. 3.14).

It is not possible to ascertain if a dysplastic ICA aneurysm is the consequence of a previous dissection or has developed in a wall that was structurally weakened by FMD. To obscure further the causality of events, we know that there is a high incidence of spontaneous dissection in arteries that bear FMD lesions and that some of these dissections will evolve into aneurysms.

As mentioned above, there is a striking difference in the incidence of dysplastic and atherosclerotic aneurysms between the large series of McCollum (USA)[32] and those of Moreau[34] and Rosset[35] (France). None of McCallum's patients was reported to have a dysplastic aneurysm, while the majority of patients in the European series had dysplastic aneurysms. There are many more reports of spontaneous dissection and FMD in the vascular literature from Europe than in the United States, and perhaps this is the reason the Europeans encounter more dysplastic ICA aneurysms. Rosset has also suggested that because CTA is the standard practice to follow up patients with ICA dissection in Europe, they are finding more dysplastic aneurysms. In fact, many of the dysplastic aneurysms described in the European series were found by CTA during follow-up studies for ICA dissection. FMD and connective tissue diseases, such

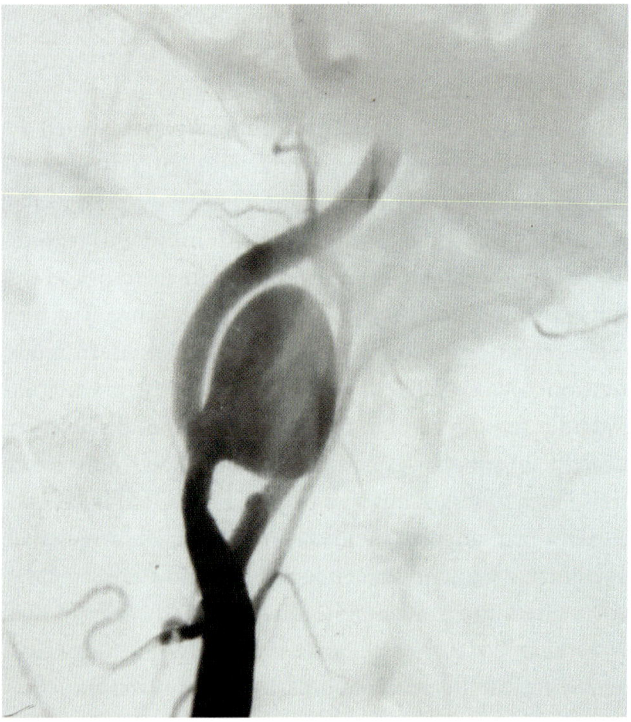

FIGURE 3.13. A dysplastic ICA aneurysm.

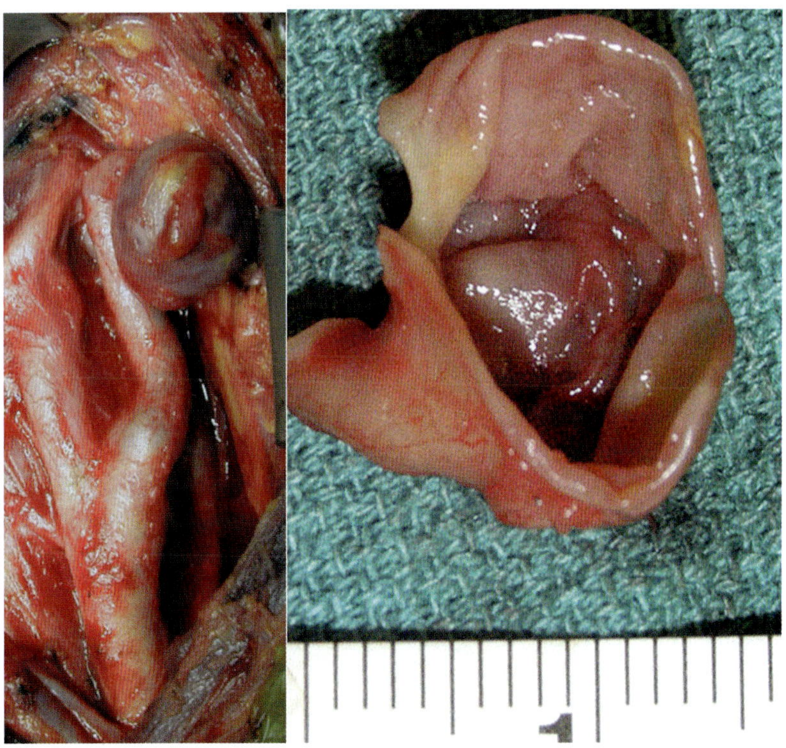

FIGURE 3.14. Operative photo of dysplastic ICA aneurysm and of its thrombus-free sac.

as Marfan's, Ehler-Danlos, and neurofibromatosis, are the causes of the majority of dysplastic ICA aneurysms.

With regard to the absence of dysplastic aneurysms in the USA series, it should be pointed out that some illustrations in McCollum's paper labeled as atherosclerotic aneurysm have the typical appearance and localization of a dysplastic aneurysm. Perhaps they were labeled as atherosclerotic because, once a dysplastic aneurysm has been present for a long time, it may develop luminal thrombus and features of atherosclerosis in its wall. These atheromatous features develop in response to the changes in flow and geometry within the aneurysm but are not its cause.

There are very few ruptures of ICA aneurysms in modern reports. Their most frequent presentation, seen in 50% of patients, is a TIA/stroke secondary to embolization.[30,36] The gender ratio in carotid aneurysms varies in different series, with males being more prevalent in some series and females in others. This is different from the much higher prevalence of males in series of aortic and peripheral aneurysms.

Nearly all (90%) primary VA aneurysms occur in its intracranial portion (V4). Of the few extracranial VA aneurysms encountered, most are secondary to trauma or dissection and they affect the most mobile part of the VA, the V3 segment.

Primary extracranial VA aneurysms are exceedingly rare with 12 such aneurysms reports encountered in the literature. We have treated seven patients with nine true extracranial primary VA aneurysms over a period of 12 years. They occurred in young individuals (mean age 38 years) with connective tissue disorders such as Ehler-Danlos (Fig. 3.15), Marfan (Fig. 3.16), and neurofibromatosis (Fig. 3.17). Three of

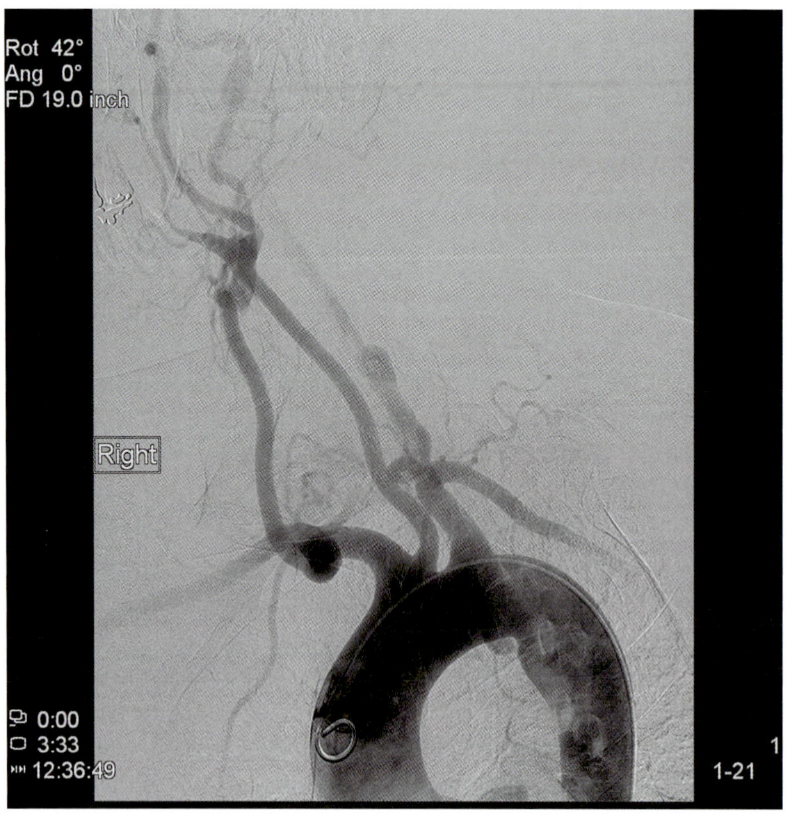

FIGURE 3.15. Bilateral vertebral aneurysms in a patient with Ehler-Danlos syndrome.

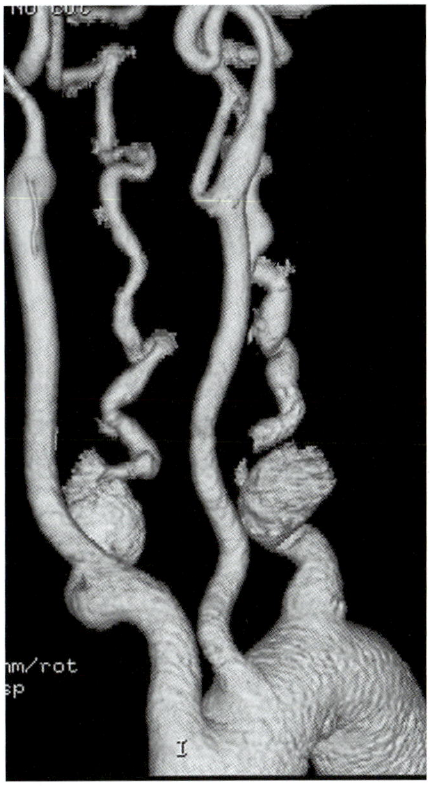

FIGURE 3.16. Bilateral VA aneurysms in a patient with Marfan's.

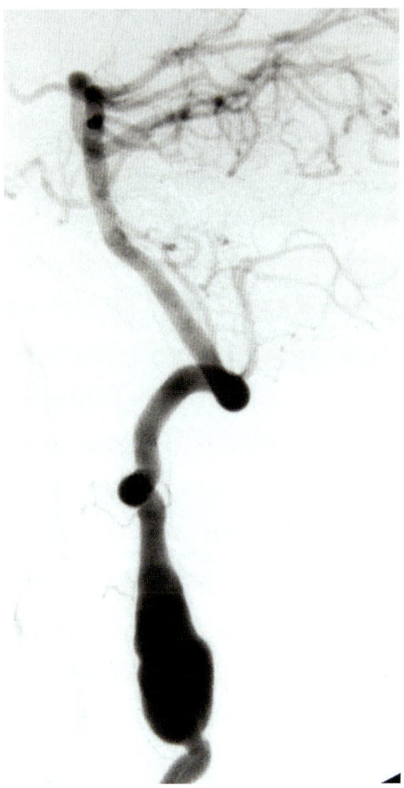

FIGURE 3.17. VA aneurysm in the V2 segment in a 15-year-old youngster with neurofibromatosis.

7 patients had a family history of aneurysm-related death secondary to a connective tissue disorder. Four of 7 patients had one or more aneurysms in other locations.

CAROTID BODY TUMORS

The published reports on carotid body tumor (CBT)[37] suggest that 6% to 10% of them are malignant (so defined by the presence of metastases). Surgeons[38] who routinely resect abnormal lymph nodes in the neighborhood of the tumor report a higher (15%) incidence of malignancy and, based upon this finding, they recommend to excise any lymph node that is enlarged or in close association with the tumor.[iv]

About 20% of CBTs are of the familiar variety and they typically present as bilateral tumors. Bilateral presentation in a patient should prompt screening of close relatives. Bilaterality (familiar type paragangliomas) (Fig. 3.18) should also prompt a CTA of the chest, neck, and abdomen, searching for additional paragangliomas, particularly within the vagus nerve (vagal paragangliomas) and in the aorto-pulmonary window[39] (Fig. 3.19).

A Schwannoma of the cervical sympathetic chain may mimic the appearance of a carotid paraganglioma[40] by being located close to the carotid bifurcation and displacing the ICA and ECA. But Schwannomas, however, do not have the hypervascularity of paragangliomas evident in CTA or arteriography.

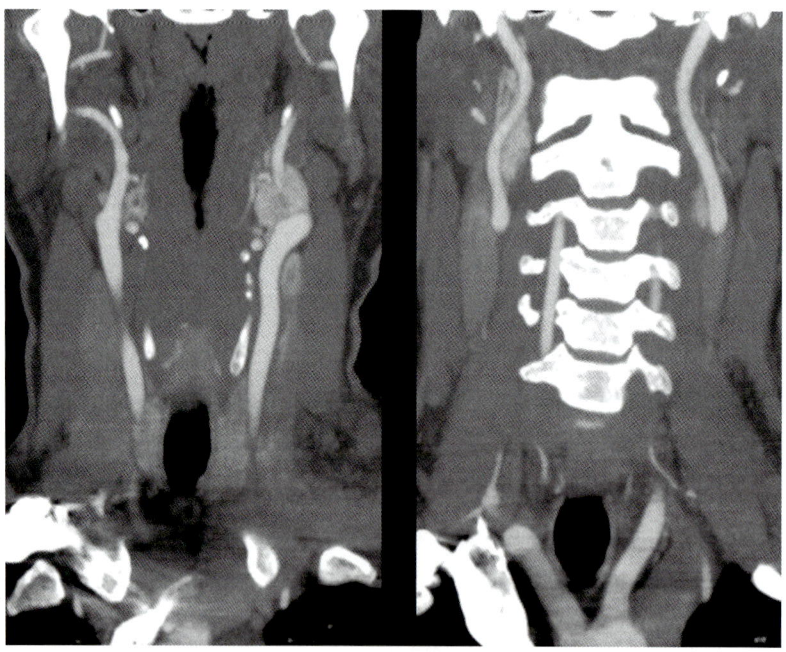

FIGURE 3.18. Bilateral carotid paraganglioma in a 24-year-old woman found on familiar screening after her father was diagnosed with familiar bilateral paraganglioma.

[iv] I do not search for or excise neighboring lymph nodes and I have not encountered malignancy in 39 CBT I have resected.

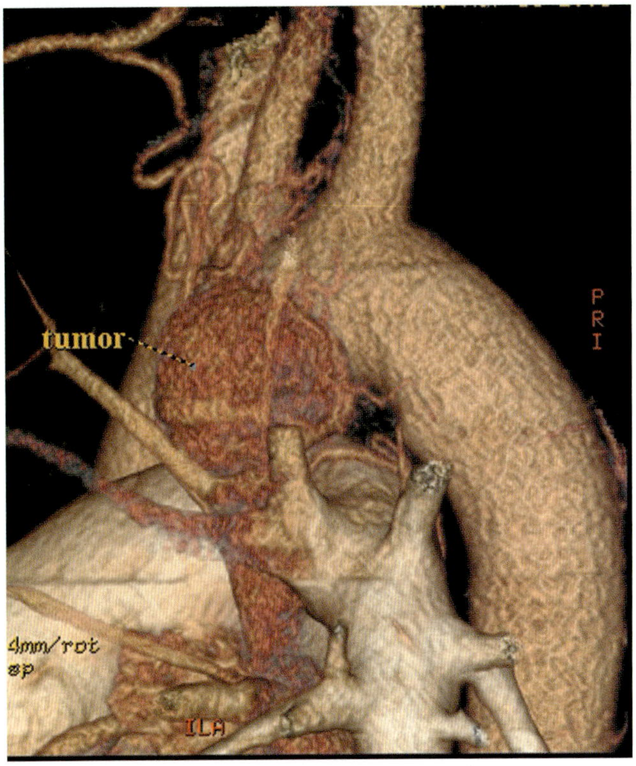

FIGURE 3.19. A paraganglioma in the aorto-pulmonary window in a patient who also had bilateral CBTs.

DYNAMIC COMPRESSION OF THE VERTEBRAL ARTERY (BOW HUNTER SYNDROME)

Dynamic compression of the VA was first described in 1927 by DeKleyn,[41] who showed in cadavers the stoppage of flow in the VA when the neck was rotated to the opposite side. Tatlow, 30 years later, injected radiopaque material in cadavers and showed that the VA was compressed at C1–C2 when the neck was rotated to the opposite side.[42] The artery returned to normal caliber when the neck was returned to the neutral position.

Dynamic compression of the VA occurs in the normal population as has been documented by Weintraub in MRA studies.[43] He showed that those individuals that had a hypoplastic VA on the side to which the neck was rotated were likely to experience dizziness or vertigo with the maneuver. The most cogent explanation was that the hypoplastic VA could not compensate the flow stoppage caused by rotation in the dominant VA. As discussed below, this latter situation is analogous to what we find in patients who have dynamic symptoms.

The VA may be compressed by either bone or tendinous slips in any of its first three segments. Before it enters the spine (V1), the VA may be compressed by the tendons of the longus colli or scalenus anticus (Fig. 3.20). The attachments of these two muscles to the transverse process of C6 diverge forming an inverted V under which the VA passes to enter the transverse process of C6.

As mentioned above, asymptomatic postural compression/occlusion of a VA with rotation of the neck is a normal finding.[43] Symptomatic compression of a single/dominant VA resulting in VBI, the so-called *bow hunter syndrome,* is an

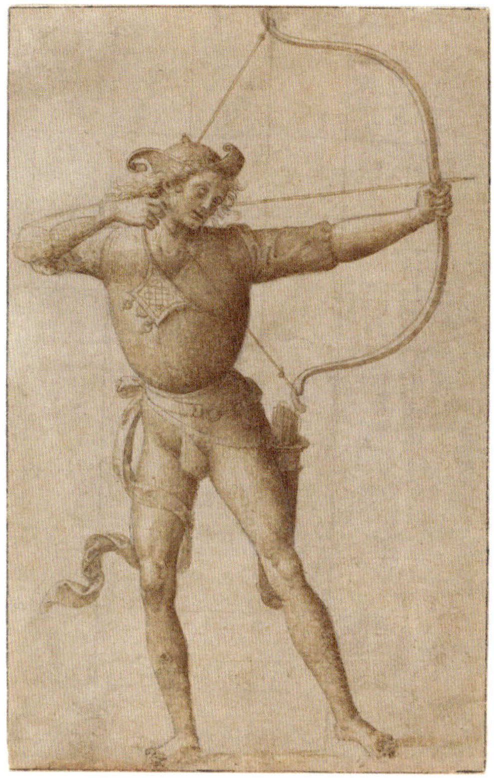

PLATE 3.1. *Figure of an Archer*, by Pietro Perugino (1450 to 1523). Two body movements in this illustration, abduction of the arm and ipsilateral rotation–extension of the neck, are capable of compressing a vertebral artery.

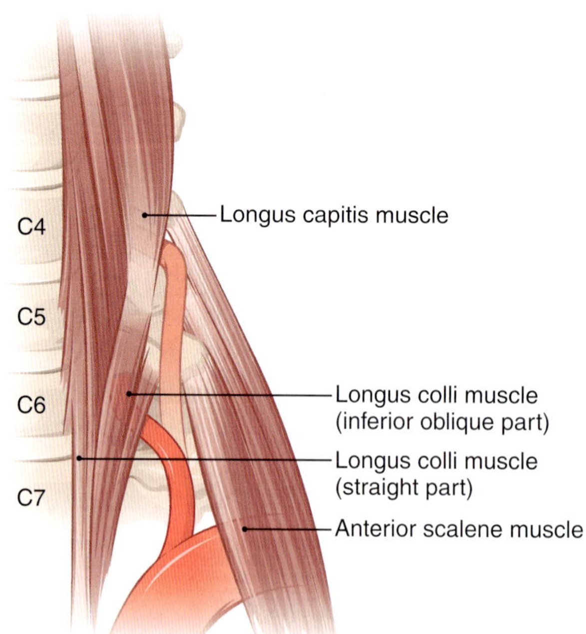

FIGURE 3.20. The VA passes under the tendons of the longus colli and scalenus anticus as it enters the spine.

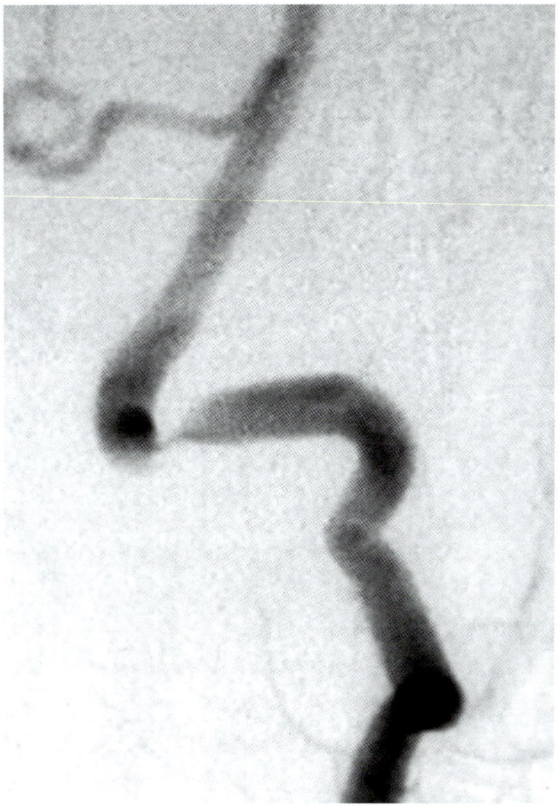

FIGURE 3.21. Compression of the VA between the occipital bone (C0) and the upper edge of the lamina of C1.

underdiagnosed condition of not infrequent occurrence. With counted exceptions, patients with bow hunter syndrome have one single functioning VA and absent posterior communicating arteries so that the occlusion of their only direct supply to the brain stem, the dominant VA, results in syncope.

While the level of compression is usually found in the V3 segment (C0–C2) (Fig. 3.21) in other cases it occurs in the V1 and V2 segments (Fig. 3.22) and even at C7 (Fig. 3.23) before the VA enters the transverse foramina of the cervical spine.[44]

While considering the mechanics of dynamic VA compression, one must bear in mind the fact that the geometry of the cervical spine changes from the supine to the standing position. When standing, the cervical spine is shortened by the weight of the head (8 to 12 lb) and the tonic contraction of the paraspinal muscles. The shortening of spinal length accentuates any kink or redundancy that may exist in the VA by changing the geometry of its bony surroundings. In fact, very few patients presenting with bow hunter syndrome experience symptoms when lying supine. When performing a dynamic arteriogram to study a patient with bow hunter syndrome, one needs to mimic this vertical axial force caused by the weight of the head: in addition to positioning the head in the trigger position (rotation–extension), one should exert axial pressure to simulate the weight of the patient's head when the patient is standing. A preferable alternative is to do the study with the patient in the vertical position strapped to the angiography table.

Dynamic arteriography proves the cause–effect relationship between rotation of the neck, stoppage of vertebral flow (seen in the arteriogram), and simultaneous appearance of symptoms.

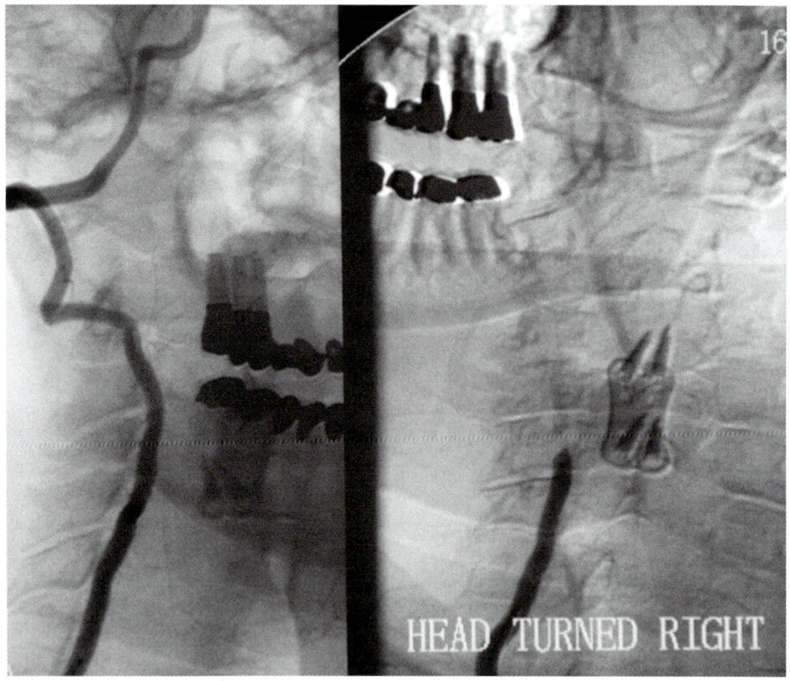

FIGURE 3.22. The VA occludes between C3 and C4 with head rotation.

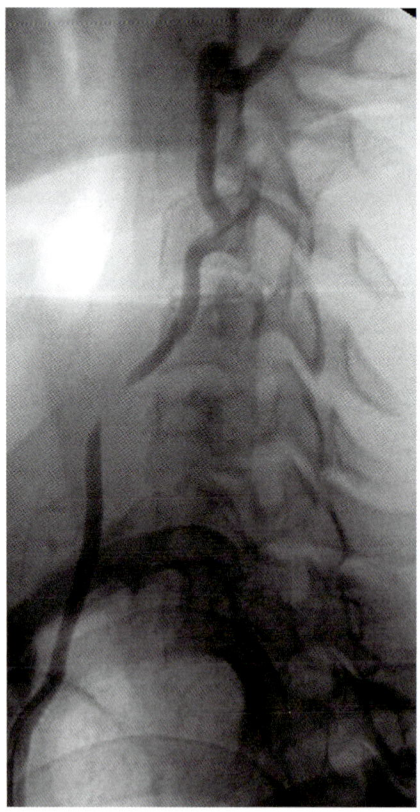

FIGURE 3.23. An unusual point of occlusion for the VA (against an enlarged transverse process of C7) with neck rotation.

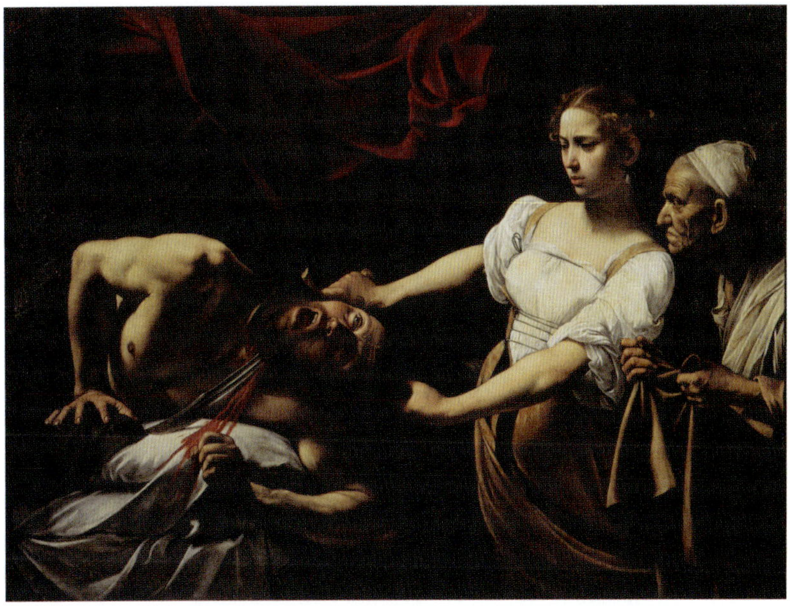

PLATE 3.2. Open carotid trauma in *Judith beheading Holofernes*, by Caravaggio "And she smote twice upon his neck with all her might, and she took away his head from him." (Judith, 13:7–8).

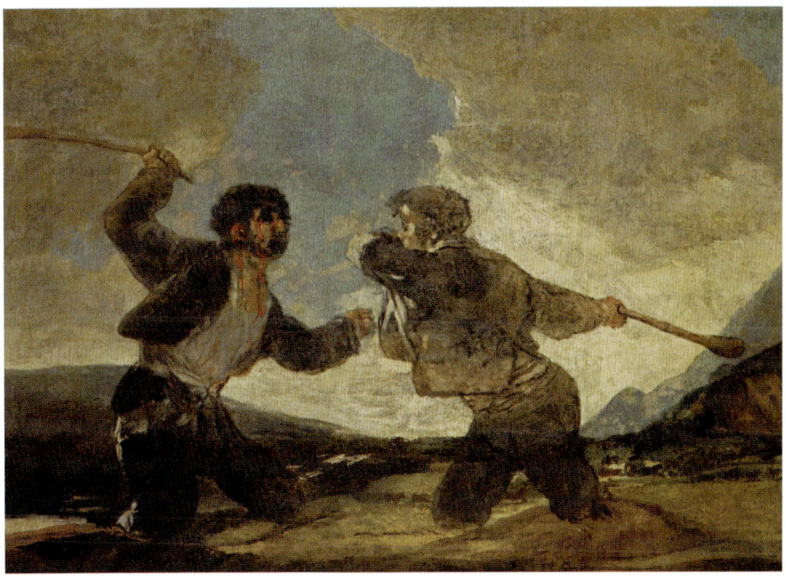

PLATE 3.3. A mechanism for blunt trauma in *Duel with cudgels*, by Goya (1746–1828). Two men with their legs buried to their knees duel to death beating each other with cudgels.

TRAUMA

Blunt anterior trauma to the chest wall can cause a dissection of the anterior SAT. A traumatic dissection of the IA generally extends into the Rt SA and Rt CCA. Two forces of disruption operate here: a direct impact on the sternum (e.g., a steering wheel in a head-on collision) and the inertial anterior displacement of the heart and

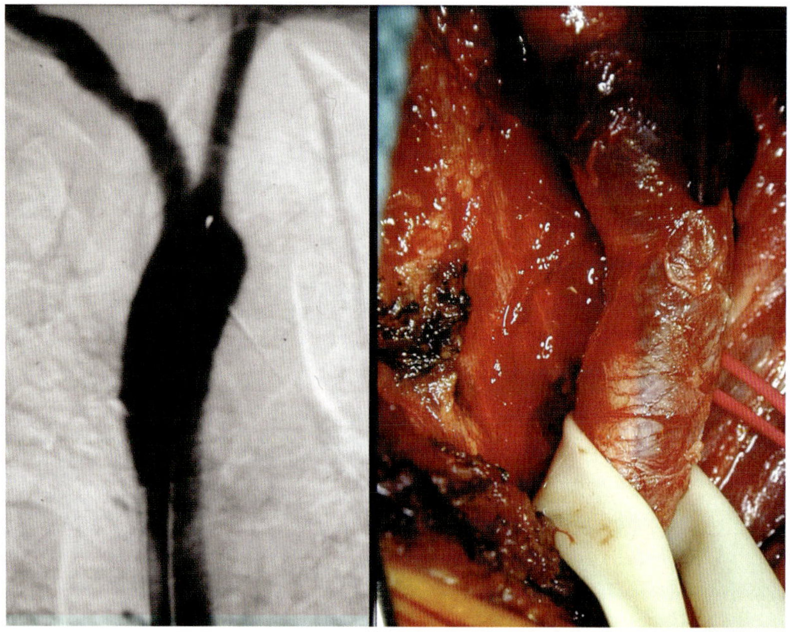

FIGURE 3.24. Following a roll-over accident this young patient presented with a left-sided hemiplegia from the occlusion of his Rt carotid system. A thrombectomy and ascending aorta–IA bypass graft reversed the neurological deficit.

ascending aorta caused by the brusque deceleration. The intramural dissection may result in thrombosis of the IA, CCA, and proximal SA (Fig. 3.24). If the outer layer ruptures in any of these dissected arteries, an aneurysm will follow (Fig. 3.11).

Blunt injuries to the carotid and vertebral arteries are uncommon and make less than 1% of all blunt trauma admissions to US hospitals. Uncommon as they are, they have a dire prognosis: 16% to 40% patients develop a stroke and between 25% and 31% die.

In *blunt trauma of the carotid artery*, the mechanism is usually a direct blow. The blow is usually external, although in some cases it can be transoral. The rare transoral trauma has been described in children who fall face down with a lollipop or a pencil in their mouth that impacts the ICA at the tonsilar fossa. A relatively recent modality of external blunt injury is attributed to the chest strap of a car's safety belt during a deceleration injury. External blunt injuries to the carotid affect more frequently the CCA than the ICA (Fig. 3.3).

Higher up in the neck, the ICA passes in front of the prominent transverse process of C1, and here, the posterior wall of the artery can be impinged by bone when the head is briskly rotated toward the opposite side. This is probably the reason why ICAs with FMD develop false aneurysms at this level (Fig. 3.25). Very rarely, a bone fragment from a fractured jaw may injure the adjacent ICA (Fig. 3.26).

Blunt vertebral artery trauma is mediated by the close relationship between the VA and the vertebral foramina through which the artery travels. A fracture of the lateral mass of a cervical vertebra or indeed a vertebral luxation or subluxation will cause sudden changes in the geometry of the osteomuscular tunnel that envelops the VA. When bone strikes the artery with sufficient force, the latter will dissect, rupture, or thrombose.

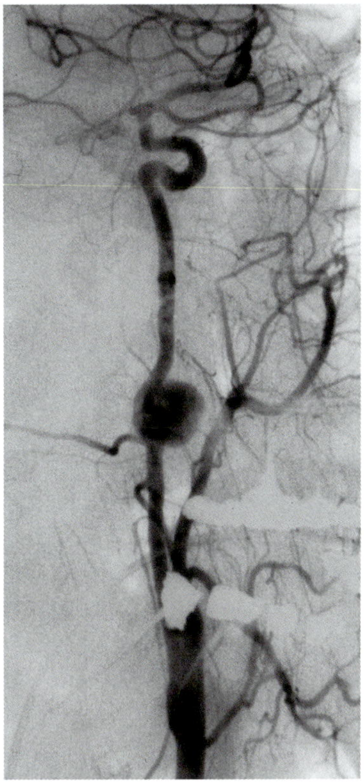

FIGURE 3.25. A dysplastic ICA aneurysm in a patient with FMD.

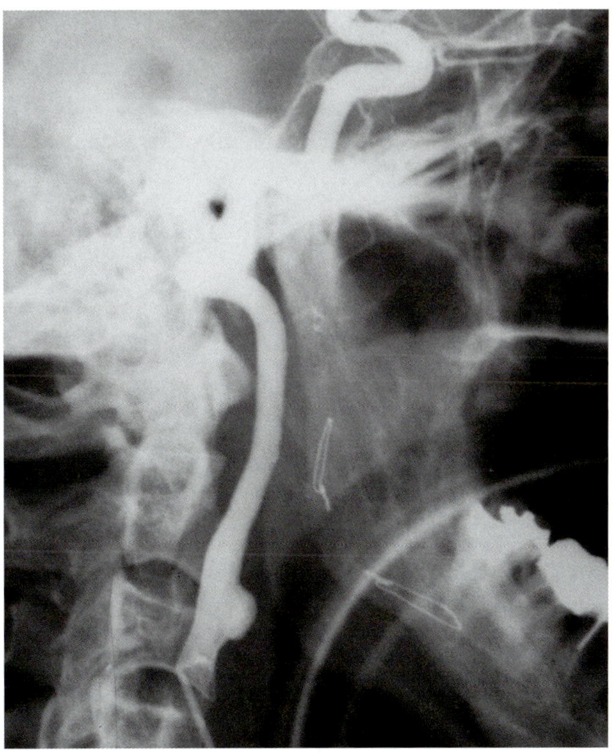

FIGURE 3.26. A small false aneurysm is seen adjacent to a fractured angle of the jaw that has been wired.

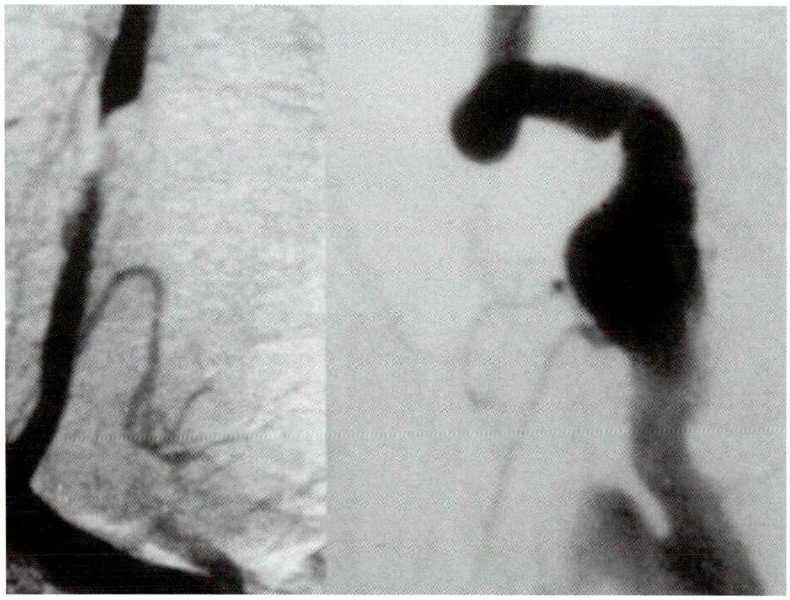

FIGURE 3.27. Osteophytic extrinsic compression (Lt) that was mistaken for an atheroma. Patient underwent angioplasty that resulted in a VA aneurysm.

A more recent etiology for traumatic aneurysms of the VA occurs when a severe VA compression (caused by an osteophyte) seen in an arteriogram is mistaken by a stenosing atheroma and a balloon angioplasty is performed. The pressurized balloon crashes the arterial wall against the rough, hard surface of the osteophyte and tears it eventually developing an aneurysm (Fig. 3.27).

When the VA is stretched beyond its normal elastic tolerance in the C1–C2 segment, it will rupture its inner layer, initiating a dissection flap, or rupture its wall. The C1–C2 joint is by far the most mobile joint of the spine: one-half of the entire range of rotation of the neck (180 degrees) takes place in it (Fig. 3.28). To

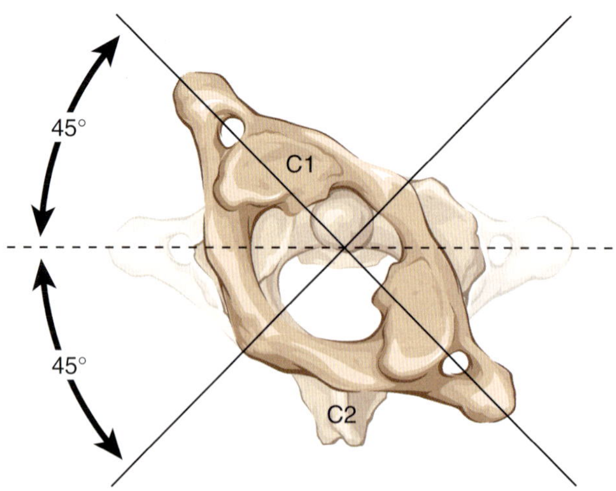

FIGURE 3.28. The arc of rotation of C1–C2 is 45 degrees to the right and to the left of the neutral position.

accommodate this wide arc (45 degrees) of rotation, the VA has an elongated loop between C1 and C2. The adventitia of the VA is attached, to the periosteum of the transverse foramina of these two vertebras. If the neck is brusquely rotated to one side, the rate of stretching of the VA between its two fixed points at C1 and C2 may exceed the elastic tolerance of the artery.[45] One can imagine the artery composed of two coaxial tubes of different tensile strength. An inner layer made up of endothelium and internal elastic lamina and a coaxial outside layer made out of media and adventitia. A sudden stretch will snap first the inner layer that contains very little elastic material. This tear of the intima and internal elastic membrane may start a dissection. If the mechanical stretching is strong enough, it may tear the wall of the VA with subsequent hemorrhage, formation of a false aneurysm, or its occlusion.

The mechanics of VA dissection, rupture, or thrombosis are generated by stretching of the artery. Like any other artery, the VA has anisotropic elastic properties. Johnson[46] tested circumferential and longitudinal strips of human VA in a tensile strength machine. The longitudinal strips ruptured with a mere 20% elongation but the circumferential strips tolerated a 20% stretch without rupture. This tells us that the mechanical failure of the VA occurs with moderate longitudinal stretching but only after a larger radial circumferential stretch. Because these authors stretched their specimens without "pre-tensing" them to their in vivo length, we can assume that the longitudinal stretch that caused the VA rupture was a mere 10%.

The position of the neck at the time of impact or stretch changes markedly the amount of elongation to which the VA is subjected. With the neck rotated,[45] a 5 g rear impact force results in 30 mm of elongation and bending of the VA. However, if the neck is in the neutral position at the time of the impact, the elongation imposed on the artery by the impact force is limited to 5 mm.

Patients with blunt injury to the carotid or vertebral arteries may not display symptoms immediately. In fact, only 50% of the patients with blunt injury to these arteries present to the emergency room with neurologic symptoms. As many as 25% of patients with blunt injuries to these arteries will develop symptoms only after an interval of neurologic normalcy.

The local lesions that can develop with blunt injury are irregularities within the lumen, disruption of the inner layer, medial hematoma or occlusion or collapse of the artery from external hemorrhage, and hematoma. An intimal flap may cause occlusion of the artery or may embolize the platelet aggregates and thrombus that form beneath it. The flap may give entry to a dissection that will progress distally and eventually decompress through a distal tear and, through the latter, embolize its contents.

A patient who is suspected to have suffered blunt injuries should undergo angiography when the following markers are present: (1) a Horner's syndrome (from involvement of the upper cervical ganglion or of the sympathetics along the arterial wall by hemorrhage or trauma); (2) presence of a neurologic deficit (after having ruled out alcohol intoxication, drugs, or hemorrhagic shock); (3) when the mechanism of injury is consistent with hyperrotation or hyperextension of the neck (motor vehicle accident); and (4) when fracture, luxation, or subluxation of a vertebra are found in the admission films. The importance of these neurologic markers has been clearly shown by Biffl.[47] Less than 1% of patients with blunt trauma admitted to an emergency room have lesions of the ICA or VA. However, among patients who have a history of blunt trauma and who exhibit any of the markers listed above, 29% to 44% of them will have an ICA or a VA injury.

US is not an adequate tool to evaluate a patient for carotid or vertebral dissection. The ICA dissections occur in the upper neck, an area difficult to insonate. In addition, the US is likely to miss small intimal injuries and the associated soft tissue trauma in the neck will cause swelling that further obscures the definition of images. US is equally useless in the evaluation of the VA for suspicion of blunt injury.

Although CTA may not always have the resolution needed to identify tiny flaps, it is a good tool to screen patients with acute cervical spine trauma. Modern multidetector CT machines can acquire in 30 seconds the data needed to display the bony and vascular abnormalities that may accompany head and neck trauma.

The CT of the brain is also a good predictor of the outcome of blunt trauma of the head and neck: if an acute infarct is seen, approximately 50% of the patients will die and 75% of them will have a permanent neurologic deficit. If the CT of the brain is normal, only 30% of the patients will develop a neurologic deficit.[47] An injury of the VA will be found in 25% of patients that present with a fracture that involves the transverse process and in 35% of those with a facet dislocation.

MRI/MRA is not generally used to visualize vascular damage in trauma patients because it is seldom immediately available in the emergency departments where these patients are attended and also because these patients often have stabilizing or ventilatory support hardware incompatible with MR protocols. If the patient has any of the markers mentioned above, an arteriogram or a CTA is indicated.

Among patients with acute cervical spine trauma who are systematically screened with MRA or CTA, 20% to 25% will show abnormalities of the VA, mostly acute occlusion or dissection, and 3% to 5% will develop a cerebellar or brain stem infarction[48–50] often lethal. Most patients presenting with a VA injury from blunt trauma will have no clinical neurologic symptoms, but the few that develop ischemic symptoms in the posterior circulation will have a morbid course. This morbid course is generally the result of the progression or embolization of the thrombus into the BA. This mechanism explains the development of VB stroke several days, even weeks, after the original blunt trauma.

A patient who has been found to have an intimal lesion in the arteriogram but has not developed a false aneurysm should be managed with heparin and followed with Coumadin, assuming there are no contraindications for the use of either drug, an unlikely situation in multiple trauma. There is consensus but no proof that dissections of the VA should be managed with heparin during the acute period and followed by Coumadin for 2 to 3 months. Symptomatic false aneurysms in either ICA or VA can be managed with stents or stent grafts and occasionally with stents and Guglielmi detachable coils inserted through the stent mesh. Surgery is reserved for those patients who have an acute symptomatic occlusion of the CA or VA, a persistent false aneurysm or a dissection that is unresponsive to anticoagulation (Fig. 3.9).

Iatrogenic trauma of the carotid or vertebral arteries is either secondary to punctures for central vein catheterization or, in the case of the VA, to accidental trauma during surgical procedures in the cervical spine.

Puncture/catheter injury is more frequent in the CCA than in the VA and it may be followed by the formation of an AV fistula or arteriovenous aneurysm because of the proximity of the corresponding venous channel: IJV or vertebral vein, respectively. In the 60s and early 70s, some AV fistulas occurred when arteriograms were done then by direct puncture of the CCA or VA. Today, when arteriograms are done by percutaneous femoral technique, the rare dissection occasionally seen in a VA following arteriography is the result of advancing the catheter and injecting into the VA proper to obtain a VB arteriogram (selective VB injections should be made in the SA proximal to the origin of the VA).

Some iatrogenic *injuries of the VA occur during spinal surgery.* It is reported that a VA injury will occur in 0.3% to 0.5% of anterior discectomies.[51,52] The favored technique for atlantoaxial fixation involves inserting a screw through the C1–C2 facet joint and carries a 8% risk of VA laceration.[53] It is obvious why these accidents may occur when we observe in some patients the marked tortuosity and elongation of their VA as it passes from one transverse process to the next. Spine surgeons have precisely defined the anatomical landmarks to be observed for safe drilling into a cervical vertebra, but the variations in the trajectory of the VA, including its extraforaminal excursions, continue to be the cause for these uncommon injuries (Fig. 3.29).

If a VA is injured during spinal surgery, the attempt to tamponade the bleeding with procoagulants and pressure may provide a temporal solution that may not always be effective. Recurrent bleeding, pseudoaneurysm, or AV fistula may follow. Attempts to ligate the artery in situ usually fail. A bleeding VA in its V2 segment is hard to access and, to add difficulty, it must be ligated above and below the site of injury. If the artery is ligated only proximally retrograde bleeding will continue from the distal VA. It must be remembered also that ligation of a VA is not necessarily a safe maneuver, particularly if the status of the opposite VA is not known. A neurosurgical review of the literature reported a 12% death following ligation[54] although in this review the inclusion of ligations done for unacceptable indications and reported a century ago probably exaggerates the risk of ligature.

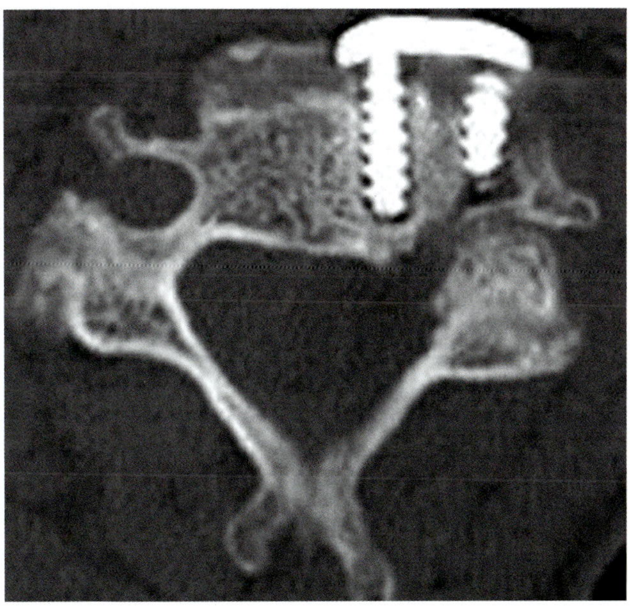

FIGURE 3.29. A screw threaded into the Rt foramen transversarium thrombosed this Lt VA. Fortunately, this VA was not a dominant one, as can be deduced by the much larger area of the contralateral foramen.

ARTERIOVENOUS FISTULA

Spontaneous AV fistula of the carotid territory is rare and most are secondary to gunshot or knife injuries. CCA to IJV fistulas, if they are of sufficient size, will manifest by a palpable thrill and the development of congestive heart failure. In the VA, trauma to the spine resulting in subluxation or fracture of a vertebra is a frequent cause of an AV fistula, because the artery is surrounded by a plexus of veins that are simultaneously injured with it: when the dislocated vertebral bone ruptures the wall of the artery, the adjacent veins are torn, and an AV fistula follows. The fistulas secondary to closed trauma occur in that part of the artery that, by being the most mobile, is most subjected to traction injury: the C1–C2 segment (Fig. 3.30). In vertebral AV fistulas, patients may experience low-flow symptoms from the effects of shunting. Shunting volume is increased by the contribution of a large reversal of flow from the distal VA into the fistulous opening.

The current common treatment of AV fistulas of the CCA is placement of an endovascular stent graft that obliterates the opening. In the VA territory, the endovascular technique of floating a detachable balloon into the venous side of the fistula[55] closes the latter and preserves the patency of the VA (Fig. 3.30). This is a better alternative than the difficulties that, in the past, accompanied the open surgical treatment of these lesions near the skull base. There is little use for stent grafts in the management of chronic AV fistula of the VA. Stent-grafting of a proximal (V1) AV fistula of the VA can be complicated by the large disparity of size (3 to 4 X) between the pre- and post-fistulous segments of the VA (Fig. 3.31). In VA fistulas of the V1 segment, one can obtain temporary control of the proximal and distal artery with endovascular

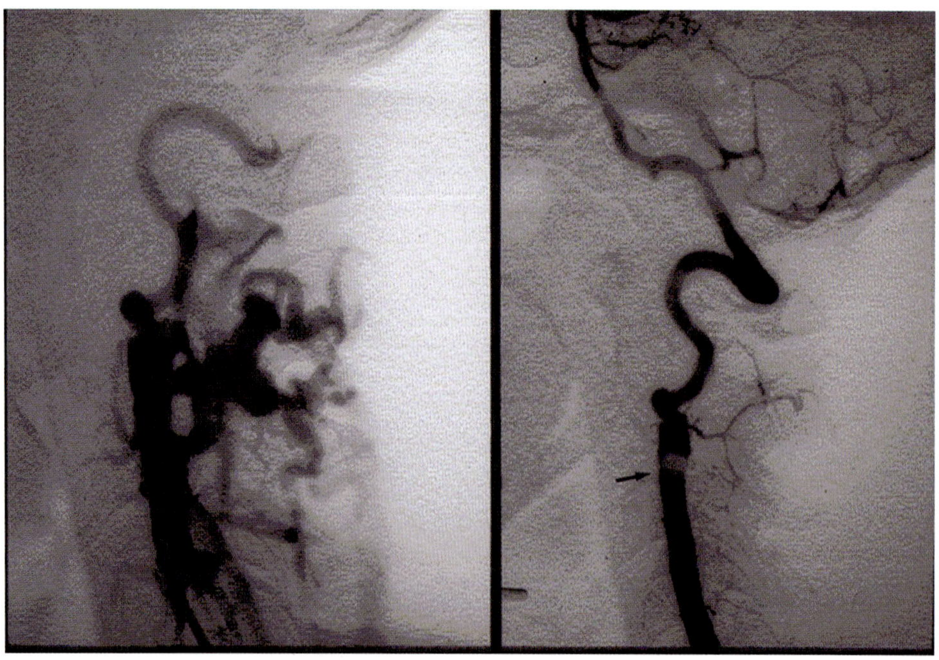

FIGURE 3.30. An AV fistula involving the V3 segment of the VA. This young boy underwent a subluxation of C1–C2 while "playing hangman" with rope around his neck over a door. The fistula was symptomatic but the patient did not have a spinal cord injury. The AV fistula was cured by parachuting a detachable balloon into its venous side.

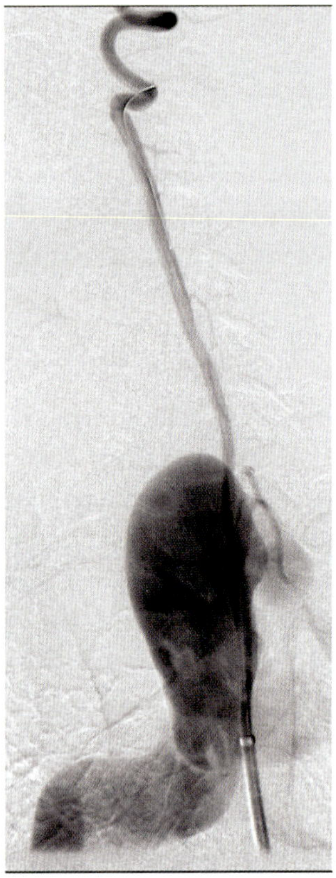

FIGURE 3.31. Early and late phase of an AV fistula of the V1 segment of the VA. The proximal VA has a diameter of 13 mm. The post-fistulous VA measures 4 mm in diameter.

balloons (Fig. 3.31) and then access the fistula through the wall of the dilated venous aneurysm to close its opening from the venous side (Fig. 3.32). If the AV fistula is located in the C1–C2 segment, navigating a stent graft up through the sharp vertebral bends at this level is problematic and risky.

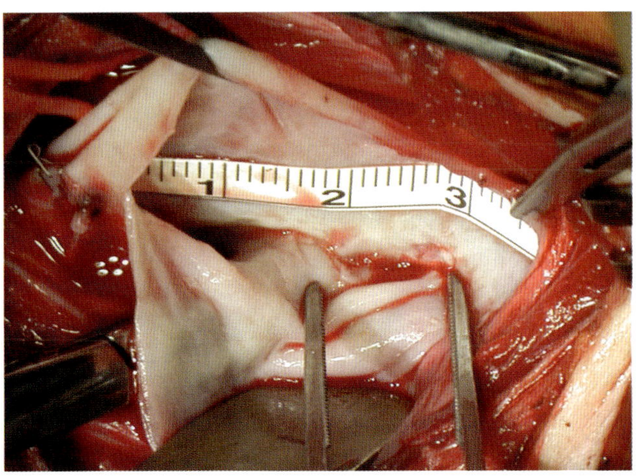

FIGURE 3.32. The aneurysm of the vertebral vein has been opened. The fistulous opening of the VA is between the jaws of the pickup forceps. The VA has been temporarily occluded above and below the fistula with catheter balloons.

RADIATION ARTERITIS

The effect of radiation on arteries is time and dose dependent. The higher the dose, the more the damage to the artery. The endothelium is the first layer affected by radiation.[56] The post-radiation lesions that develop in the carotid and vertebral arteries have the same composition as atherosclerotic lesions but they develop in places that are usually spared by atheromatous plaques, such as the CCA, and the infrapetrosal segment of the ICA. In the VA, its V1 segment is involved when patients receive radiation for treatment of head and neck cancer. Rarely the intraspinal segment (V2, V3) may also be affected.

Although irradiation may cause fibrous arterial stenosis without the traditional heterogeneous composition of an atherosclerotic plaque, most of the atheromatous disease that develops in radiated arteries is of heterogeneous composition and often of atopical location. The manifestations of radiation in the CA and VA may appear as early as 1 year and as late as 20 years after the exposure to radiation and they are usually limited to the radiated field. As expected, the effects of radiation in this area involve also the smaller arteries within the area, a situation that can only aggravate the consequences of thrombosis of the large artery (CCA, ICA) because the collateral circulation has also been decimated.

In the carotid artery, radiation arteritis may follow a different and dramatic pathway: rupture of the carotid artery a month or two after radiotherapy and radical resection of head and neck cancer. On the other hand, a carotid blowout is exceptionally rare in patients who have had only radiation. It is likely that the rupture of the wall of the CCA results from the compounding effect of ionizing damage to the arterial wall and the surgical dissection that does away with the periadventitial blood vessels that supply 75% of this wall. Leaving aside the rare occurrence of an early blowout, in the vast majority of cases the manifestations of radiation arteritis appear 1 to 20 years after exposure, resemble atherosclerotic plaques, and result in the same clinical consequences (stroke). The time taken for a carotid artery to display the consequences of radiation may well be even beyond 20 years, but the limited life expectancy of patients undergoing radiation of the neck for cancer does not permit to test this proposition.

Linear follow-up of atherosclerotic plaques in patients with cancer of the head and neck showed that those who were radiated had a statically significant increase in the thickness of their plaques when compared to those who did not have radiation.[57] This suggests that radiation may not only generate atherosclerotic-like lesions in the carotid and vertebral arteries but also act as an accelerator of preexisting disease in them.

To summarize, the arterial damage caused by radiation may appear many years after treatment and is manifested by exuberant atherosclerotic lesions that often extend into locations of unusual topography.

VERTEBRAL ARTERY DISSECTION AND CHIROPRACTIC MANIPULATION

Our extracranial arteries are, mechanically, viscoelastic tubes. As such, when stretched slowly (as when we rotate our neck 90 degrees to look sideways) their walls experience much lower mechanical stresses than when their wall is stretched brusquely (e.g., snapping the neck sideways in a motor vehicle accident).

The chiropractic practice of "high impact" rotation of the neck has been identified as being the cause of VA dissections and subsequent, often fatal, strokes. This was first reported in 1947 by Pratt-Thompson who found thrombosis of the BA and the PICA in two patients who developed a VB stroke after chiropractic manipulation. It has been shown experimentally that even a modest elongation of 10% can rupture the wall of the VA. Ivancic[45] demonstrated that a rear impact will caused a much larger elongation of the VA if the head had been rotated before the impact.

The incidence of VB stroke in the chiropractic literature, based on self-reporting, is very low: 1/1.3 million to 1/400,000 treatment sessions. Population-based control studies[58] deriving data from admission codes for VB stroke and billing codes for chiropractic manipulation showed a higher incidence of 1.3 strokes in 100,000 treatment sessions. However low this incidence of stroke may be, the outcome of VB stroke after neck manipulation is dire: 52% of patients will have a permanent neurologic deficit and 5% to 18% will die.[59–61] The cause–effect relationship is suggested by the timing of the development of the posterior circulation infarct following chiropractic manipulation. The population-based study mentioned above[58] also showed that young patients (<45 years) admitted with a neurological deficit following VA dissection or occlusion were five times more likely than matched controls to have visited a chiropractor for cervical pain in the week before.

A mollified explanation about the role of the chiropractic manipulation posits that in some cases it might have extended a preexisting smaller injury. Neck pain, the usual presentation of spontaneous VA dissection, is often the reason a patient goes to the chiropractor. The neck pain often follows an injury, not infrequently a sport injury (Fig. 3.5), or it may appear in an individual with a connective tissue disorder. The addition of high impact manipulation may cause the morbid extension of what might have been a mere incipient dissection of the VA in the trauma cases or the beginning of a dissection in patients with elastic disorders (Marfan, Ehler-Danlos, etc.).

THE INVENTION OF CAROTIDYNIA

The term "carotidynia" was first introduced by Fay[62] in 1927 to describe tenderness in the neck over the carotid artery. Oddly enough, what began as the name of a symptom became a distinct pathological entity defined as unilateral pain and tenderness over the carotid artery. Carotidynia was an exotic but not infrequently reported diagnosis 40 years ago. It was described as a self-limiting inflammatory event of unknown etiology, lasting a few weeks, manifested by pain originating in a carotid sheath that, on the other hand, did not appear thickened with inflammation in the few patients that had imaging studies.

Reviewing the cases reported in the literature, Biousse[63] pointed out gross inconsistencies in the presentation of pain, in the degree of tenderness of the carotid to palpation, and in the duration of their symptoms. Only a few of the many cases reported had undergone imaging studies. And in some of the few imaging studies available other arterial lesions were seen, such as dissections, cystic medial necrosis, or intraplaque hemorrhage, that could have caused the neck tenderness in question.

Biousse has sensibly proposed that the neck pain and/or carotid tenderness with which these patients present is probably a local expression of a number of vascular (dissection, intraplaque hemorrhage) and non-vascular (migraine, lymphadenitis, etc.)

entities. He sensibly concluded that the term "carotidynia" does not represent a distinct pathological entity and should be abandoned.

REFERENCES

1. Tomandl BF, Klotz E, Handschu R, et al. Comprehensive imaging of ischemic stroke with multisection CT. *Radiographics.* 2003;23:565–592.
2. Berguer R, Sieggreen MY, Lazo A, Hodakowski GT. The silent brain infarct in carotid surgery. *J Vasc Surg.* 1986;3:442–447.
3. Culebras A, Kase CS, Masdeu JC, et al. Practice guidelines for the use of imaging in transient ischemic attacks and acute stroke. A report of the Stroke Council, American Heart Association. *Stroke.* 1997;28:1480–1497.
4. Schellinger PD, Richter G, Kohrmann M, Dorfler A. Noninvasive angiography (magnetic resonance and computed tomography) in the diagnosis of ischemic cerebrovascular disease. Techniques and clinical applications. *Cerebrovasc Dis.* 2007;24(suppl 1):16–23.
5. Glagov S, Bassiouny HS, Sakaguchi Y, Goudet CA, Vito RP. Mechanical determinants of plaque modeling, remodeling and disruption. *Atherosclerosis.* 1997;131(suppl):S13–S14.
6. Russell DA, Wijeyaratne SM, Gough MJ. Changes in carotid plaque echomorphology with time since a neurologic event. *J Vasc Surg.* 2007;45:367–372.
7. Biasi GM, Froio A, Diethrich EB, et al. Carotid plaque echolucency increases the risk of stroke in carotid stenting: the imaging in carotid angioplasty and risk of stroke (ICAROS) study. *Circulation.* 2004;110:756–762.
8. Sabetai MM, Tegos TJ, Nicolaides AN, et al. Hemispheric symptoms and carotid plaque echomorphology. *J Vasc Surg.* 2000;31:39–47.
9. Mettinger KL. Fibromuscular dysplasia and the brain. II. Current concept of the disease. *Stroke.* 1982;13:53–58.
10. Mettinger KL, Ericson K. Fibromuscular dysplasia and the brain. I. Observations on angiographic, clinical and genetic characteristics. *Stroke.* 1982;13:46–52.
11. Slovut DP, Olin JW. Fibromuscular dysplasia. *N Engl J Med.* 2004;350:1862–1871.
12. Redekop GJ. Extracranial carotid and vertebral artery dissection: a review. *Can J Neurol Sci.* 2008;35:146–152.
13. Chaves C, Estol C, Esnaola MM, et al. Spontaneous intracranial internal carotid artery dissection: report of 10 patients. *Arch Neurol.* 2002;59:977–981.
14. Fullerton HJ, Johnston SC, Smith WS. Arterial dissection and stroke in children. *Neurology.* 2001;57:1155–1160.
15. Calvet D, Boutouyrie P, Touze E, Laloux B, Mas J-L, Laurent S. Increased stiffness of the carotid wall material in patients with spontaneous cervical artery dissection. *Stroke.* 2004;35:2078–2082.
16. Boutouyrie P, Germain DP, Fiessinger J-N, Laloux B, Perdu J, Laurent S. Increased carotid wall stress in vascular Ehlers-Danlos syndrome. *Circulation.* 2004;109:1530–1535.
17. Dittrich R, Heidbreder A, Rohsbach D, et al. Connective tissue and vascular phenotype in patients with cervical artery dissection. *Neurology.* 2007;68:2120–2124.
18. Guillon B, Peynet J, Bertrand M, Benslamia L, Bousser M-G, Tzourio C. Do extracellular-matrix-regulating enzymes play a role in cervical artery dissection? *Cerebrovasc Dis.* 2007;23:299–303.
19. Stemper BD, Yoganandan N, Pintar FA. Methodology to study intimal failure mechanics in human internal carotid arteries. *J Biomech.* 2005;38:2491–2496.
20. Pelkonen O, Tikkakoski T, Pyhtinen J, Sotaniemi K. Cerebral CT and MRI findings in cervicocephalic artery dissection. *Acta Radiol.* 2004;45:259–265.
21. Paciaroni M, Caso V, Agnelli G. Magnetic resonance imaging, magnetic resonance and catheter angiography for diagnosis of cervical artery dissection. *Front Neurol Neurosci.* 2005;20:102–118.
22. Vertinsky AT, Schwartz NE, Fischbein NJ, Rosenberg J, Albers GW, Zaharchuk G. Comparison of multidetector ct angiography and MR imaging of cervical artery dissection. *Am J Neuroradiol.* 2008;29:1753–1760.
23. Baumgartner RW, Bogousslavsky J. Clinical manifestations of carotid dissection. *Front Neurol Neurosci.* 2005;20:70–76.
24. Lucas C, Moulin T, Deplanque D, Tatu L, Chavot D. Stroke patterns of internal carotid artery dissection in 40 patients. *Stroke.* 1998;29:2646–2648.
25. Benninger DH, Georgiadis D, Kremer C, Studer A, Nedeltchev K, Baumgartner RW. Mechanism of ischemic infarct in spontaneous carotid dissection. *Stroke.* 2004;35:482–485.
26. Touze E, Gauvrit JY, Moulin T, Meder JF, Bracard S, Mas JL. Risk of stroke and recurrent dissection after a cervical artery dissection: a multicenter study. *Neurology.* 2003;61:1347–1351.

27. Schievink WI. Spontaneous dissection of the carotid and vertebral arteries. *N Engl J Med.* 2001;345: 467–467.
28. Bassetti C, Carruzzo A, Sturzenegger M, Tuncdogan E. Recurrence of cervical artery dissection. A prospective study of 81 patients. *Stroke.* 1996;10:1804–1807.
29. Menon R, Kerry S, Norris JW, Markus HS. Treatment of cervical artery dissection: a systematic review and meta-analysis. *J Neurol Neurosurg Psychiatr.* 2008;79:1122–1127.
30. Faggioli GL, Freyrie A, Stella A, et al. Extracranial internal carotid artery aneurysms: results of a surgical series with long-term follow-up. *J Vasc Surg.* 1996;23:587–594; discussion 594–585.
31. de Jong KP, Zondervan PE, van Urk H. Extracranial carotid artery aneurysms. *Eur J Vasc Surg.* 1989;3:557–562.
32. McCollum CH, Wheeler WG, Noon GP, DeBakey ME. Aneurysms of the extracranial carotid artery. Twenty-one years' experience. *Am J Surg.* 1979;137:196–200.
33. El-Sabrout R, Cooley DA. Extracranial carotid artery aneurysms: Texas Heart Institute experience. *J Vasc Surg.* 2000;31:702–712.
34. Moreau P, Albat B, Thevenet A. Surgical treatment of extracranial internal carotid artery aneurysm. *Ann Vasc Surg.* 1994;8:409–416.
35. Rosset E, Albertini JN, Magnan PE, Ede B, Thomassin JM, Branchereau A. Surgical treatment of extracranial internal carotid artery aneurysms. *J Vasc Surg.* 2000;31:713–723.
36. Zwolak RM, Whitehouse WM Jr, et al. Atherosclerotic extracranial carotid artery aneurysms. *J Vasc Surg.* 1984;1:415–422.
37. Dias Da Silva A, O'Donnell S, Gillespie D, Goff J, Shriver C, Rich N. Malignant carotid body tumor: a case report. *J Vasc Surg.* 2000;32:821–823.
38. Kruger AJ, Walker PJ, Foster WJ, Jenkins JS, Boyne NS, Jenkins J. Important observations made managing carotid body tumors during a 25-year experience. *J Vasc Surg.* 2010;52:1518–1523.
39. Vandy FC, Sisk G, Berguer R. Synchronous carotid body and thoracic paraganglioma associated with a germline sdhc mutation. *J Vasc Surg.* 2011;53:805–807.
40. Uzun L, Ugur MB, Ozdemir H. Cervical sympathetic chain schwannoma mimicking a carotid body tumor: a case report. *Tumori.* 2005;91:84–86.
41. DeKleyn A, Nieuwenhuyse P. Schwindelanfalle und nystagmus bei einer bestimmten stellung des kopfes. *Acta Otolaryngol.* 1927;11:155–157.
42. Tissington Tatlow WF, Bammer HG. Syndrome of vertebral artery compression. *Neurology.* 1957;7:331–340.
43. Weintraub MI, Khoury A. Critical neck position as an independent risk factor for posterior circulation stroke. A magnetic resonance angiographic analysis. *J Neuroimaging* 1995;5:16–22.
44. Lee V, Riles TS, Stableford J, Berguer R. Two case presentations and surgical management of bow hunter's syndrome associated with bony abnormalities of the c7 vertebra. *J Vasc Surg.* 2011;53:1381–1385.
45. Ivancic PC, Ito S, Tominaga Y, Carlson EJ, Rubin W, Panjabi MM. Effect of rotated head posture on dynamic vertebral artery elongation during simulated rear impact. *Clin Biomech* 2006;21:213–220.
46. Johnson CP, How T, Scraggs M, West CR, Burns J. A biomechanical study of the human vertebral artery with implications for fatal arterial injury. *Forensic Sci Int.* 2000;109:169–182.
47. Biffl WL, Moore EE, Offner PJ, Burch JM. Blunt carotid and vertebral arterial injuries. *World J Surg.* 2001;25:1036–1043.
48. Friedman D, Flanders A, Thomas C, Millar W. Vertebral artery injury after acute cervical spine trauma: rate of occurrence as detected by MR angiography and assessment of clinical consequences. *Am J Roentgenol.* 1995;164:443–447; discussion 448–449.
49. Willis BK, Greiner F, Orrison WW, Benzel EC. The incidence of vertebral artery injury after midcervical spine fracture or subluxation. *Neurosurgery.* 1994;34:435–441; discussion 441–432.
50. Giacobetti FB, Vaccaro AR, Bos-Giacobetti MA, et al. Vertebral artery occlusion associated with cervical spine trauma. A prospective analysis. *Spine.* 1997;22:188–192.
51. Burke JP, Gerszten PC, Welch WC. Iatrogenic vertebral artery injury during anterior cervical spine surgery. *Spine.* 2005;5:508–514; discussion 514.
52. Inamasu J, Guiot BH. Vascular injury and complication in neurosurgical spine surgery. *Acta Neurochir (Wien).* 2006;148:375–387.
53. Madawi AA, Casey AT, Solanki GA, Tuite G, Veres R, Crockard HA. Radiological and anatomical evaluation of the atlantoaxial transarticular screw fixation technique. *J Neurosurg.* 1997;86:961–968.
54. Shintani A, Zervas NT. Consequence of ligation of the vertebral artery. *J Neurosurg.* 1972;36:447–450.
55. Berguer R, Joel Feldman J, Wilner H, Lazo A. Arteriovenous vertebral fistulae: cure by combination of operation and detachable intravascular baloon. *Ann Surg.* 1982;196:65–68.
56. Fajardo LF, Lee A. Rupture of major vessels after radiation. *Cancer.* 1975;36:904–913.
57. Moritz MW, Higgins RF, Jacobs JR. Duplex imaging and incidence of carotid radiation injury after high-dose radiotherapy for tumors of the head and neck. *Arch Surg.* 1990;125:1181–1183.
58. Rothwell DM, Bondy SJ, Williams JI. Chiropractic manipulation and stroke: a population-based case-control study. *Stroke.* 2001;32:1054–1060.

59. Assendelft WJ, Bouter LM, Knipschild PG. Complications of spinal manipulation: a comprehensive review of the literature. *J Fam Pract.* 1996;42:475–480.
60. Frisoni GB, Anzola GP. Vertebrobasilar ischemia after neck motion. *Stroke.* 1991;22:1452–1460.
61. Reuter U, Hamling M, Kavuk I, Einhaupl KM, Schielke E. Vertebral artery dissections after chiropractic neck manipulation in germany over three years. *J Neurol.* 2006;253:724–730.
62. Fay T. Atypical facial neurlgia. *Arch Neurol Psyhchiat.* 1927;18:309–315.
63. Biousse V, Bousser MG. The myth of carotidynia. *Neurology.* 1994;44:993–995.

CHAPTER 4

Operations on the Supraortic Trunks

The supraaortic trunks may be repaired directly through a trans-sternal approach and remotely through cervical incisions.

TRANS-THORACIC REPAIRS: THE UPPER MIDSTERNOTOMY

The advantages of the upper midsternotomy[i] over the conventional full sternotomy are straightforward: the lower half of the thorax remains splinted by the intact lower sternum and this decreases postoperative pain (smaller sternal incision and immobility of the sternal edges) and facilitates the mechanics of respiration.

The incision starts with a 1 inch cut along the anterior tendon of the sternomastoid to the suprasternal notch and, from there, it follows the midline of the sternum for three segments (Fig. 4.1). The fibrous ligaments behind the notch are cut. The upper sternum is split with the oscillating saw to the level of T3–T4, at which level the saw is rotated to make a notch on the right half of the sternum without fully dividing it. This notch will result in a subperiosteal fracture when the sternal edges are spread in small steps with a Touffier or a pediatric Finochietto retractor.

The two lightly overlapping lobes of the thymus are separated and the thymic and thyroid ima veins draining into the brachiocephalic vein are divided. The brachiocephalic vein is dissected for 4 cm on both sides of the midline.

As the retractor is gently opened the amount of stretching that is being imposed on the brachiocephalic vein is checked visually and by palpation of the vein. Failure to do so may result in a tear of the junction of the brachiocephalic vein with the superior vena cava, a situation that is awkward to control and repair.

Below the thymus the pericardium is tented upward and opened exposing the ascending aorta. Individual sutures slung over the sternal retractor keep the pericardial edges open. Some of the fat surrounding the ascending aorta is excised to provide a better grip for the partial exclusion clamp later. The intended site for

---

[i] In 1983, during a sternotomy for an ascending aorta to IA bypass, a poorly controlled oscillating saw veered to the right and cut the right hemisternum at the level of T4. While pondering the consequences of this mishap I placed a small pediatric sternal retractor in the upper half of the sternum and noted that through the V-shaped opening the entire ascending aorta could be exposed as well as it would have been through a full sternotomy. Since then I have used a partial midsternotomy for all reconstructions based on the ascending aorta except in the rare instances where there was a need to access the left SA as well.

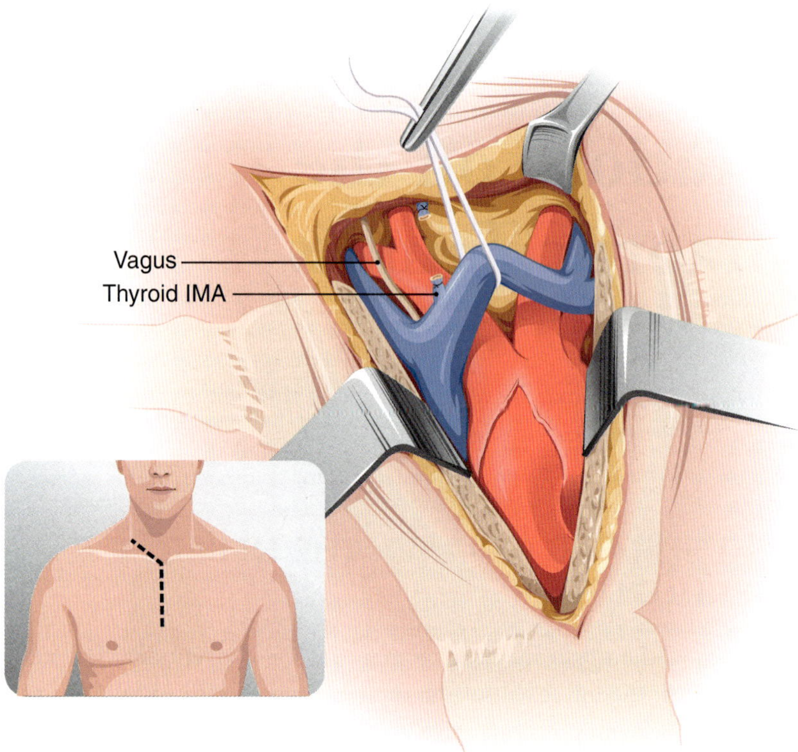

FIGURE 4.1. An upper midsternotomy exposes the ascending aorta.

exclusion clamping is inspected and palpated for the presence of atheroma or calcification (the preoperative CTA should have established the presence of calcification or thrombus at this site).

The dissection proceeds over the trunk of the IA up to its bifurcation into the Rt CCA and SA. In order to expose the full length of the IA, it is necessary to divide the sternothyroid and the sternohyoid muscles. When dissecting the bifurcation of the IA, care is taken to protect the recurrent nerve in two locations: where it hugs the lower wall of the SA origin and where the nerve is close to the posterior wall of the origin of the CCA as it crosses behind it on its medial course toward the thyroid. At this latter, and less publicized, site the recurrent nerve may be injured while circling the origin of the CCA with a right angle clamp.

Once the origins of the Rt CCA and Rt SA are isolated one can proceed with partial-exclusion clamping of the ascending aorta[1] for the proximal anastomosis of the bypass (Fig. 4.2). *Clamping of the ascending aorta* is done without heparinizing the patient and having reduced the mean aortic pressure to 80 mmHg. The clamp is a Lemole-Strong, designed in a way that protects the jaws from slipping away from the aorta. The clamp excludes only an edge of aorta large enough to make a safe anastomosis. When the clamp is closed on the aorta attention should be paid to any qualitative or quantitative change in the radial artery waveform signaling a ventricular outflow obstruction caused by too large a bite on the ascending aorta.

The excluded aorta is aspirated with a 19-gauge needle till it puckers to prove the closure of the clamp is complete. The aorta is then opened longitudinally and a small

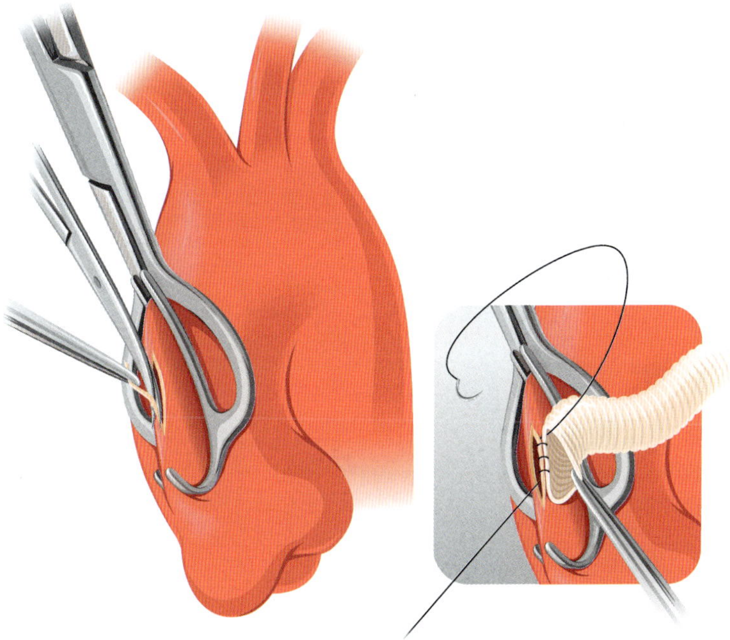

FIGURE 4.2. Partial exclusion clamping of the ascending aorta with a Lemole-Strong clamp.

sliver of wall is removed from one side. The graft selected to replace the IA artery is a #10 tube with its proximal end cut slanted to result in an anastomosis that is tangent to the ascending aorta. It is sutured with 4-0 polypropylene. Prior to tying it, any slack in its loops is corrected tenting them with a fine nerve hook. Before testing the anastomosis, the head of the patient is placed in 15 degrees of Trendelenburg to ensure that any air that could be trapped in the excluded aorta is bled out through the graft and will not escape to the more distal portion of the aortic arch.

The bypass graft is tended over the brachiocephalic vein into the proximity of the exposed bifurcation of the IA artery. Some descriptions of this technique have placed the IA bypass behind the brachiocephalic vein. That would be acceptable if the bypass had taken origin from the same site as the native IA. But the origin of the bypass is 6 to 7 cm proximal, and anterior to, to that of the IA (Fig. 4.3). A bypass placed under the brachiocephalic vein may compress the latter and itself kink at that level.

For the *distal anastomosis*, the patient is heparinized and the Rt CCA and the Rt SA are clamped. The IA is clamped in a portion devoid of calcified plaque. The artery is divided 10 mm below its bifurcation where the end of the prosthetic bypass is anastomosed to the distal rim of IA before its bifurcation (Figs. 4.4 and 4.5).

The most common supraaortic reconstruction is an aorto-distal IA bypass with a Lt CCA branch (Fig. 4.6). When a branch is needed to revascularize the left common carotid, a #8 straight graft would have been attached to the left wall of the #10 main graft beforehand. Occasionally, the bypass arising from the ascending aorta needs to reach the carotid bifurcation in one or both sides.

The choice of a #10 prosthesis for the ascending aorta–IA bypass with a #8 side branch to the Lt CCA (Fig. 4.7) is better than to use a commercial bifurcation graft,

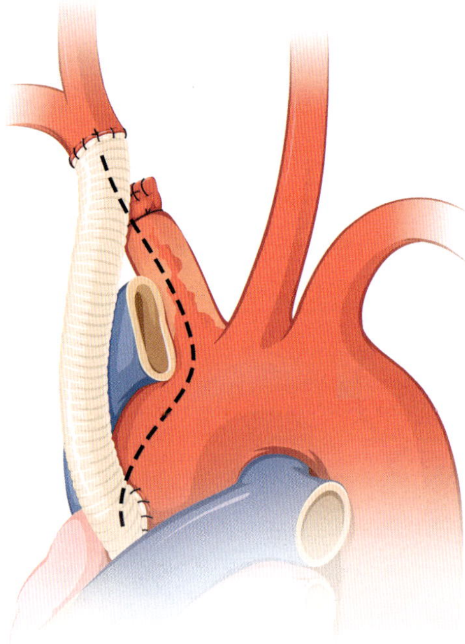

FIGURE 4.3. Schematic showing that for the bypass graft to have a straight and unimpeded course it must be placed in front of the brachiocephalic vein.

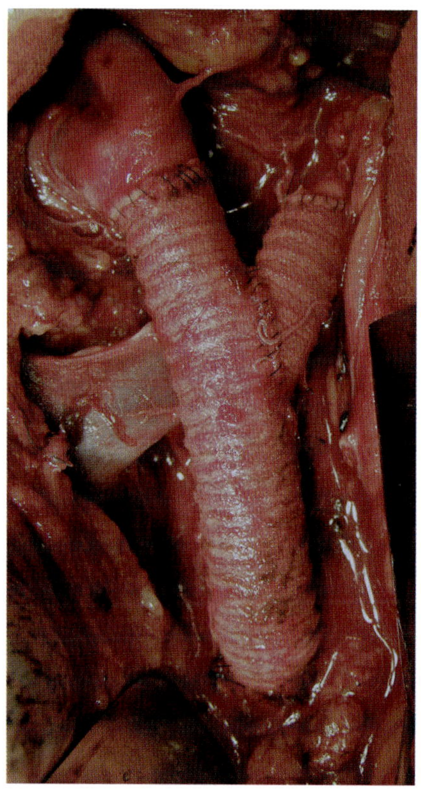

FIGURE 4.4. A completed aorto-distal IA bypass.

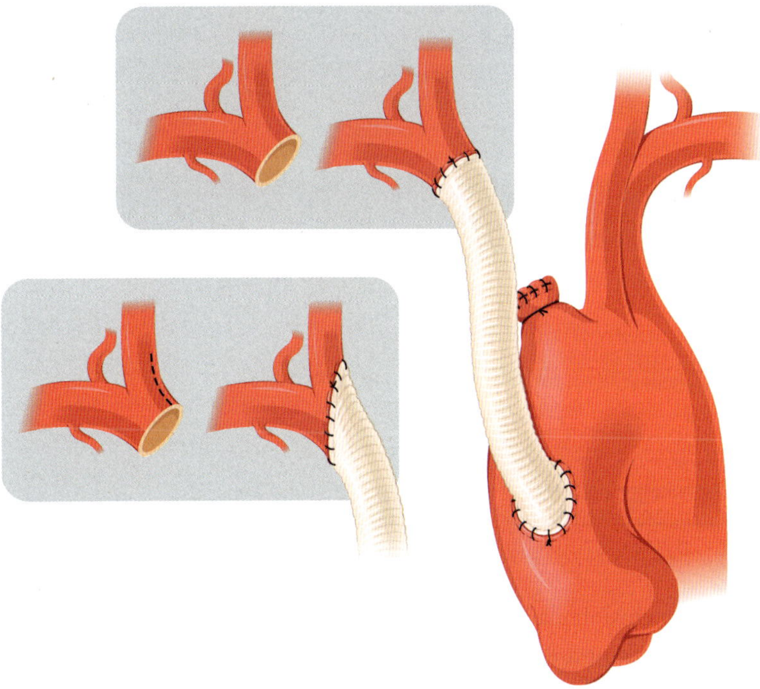

FIGURE 4.5. The distal anastomosis is fashioned extending it to the artery that bears the heaviest burden of plaque.

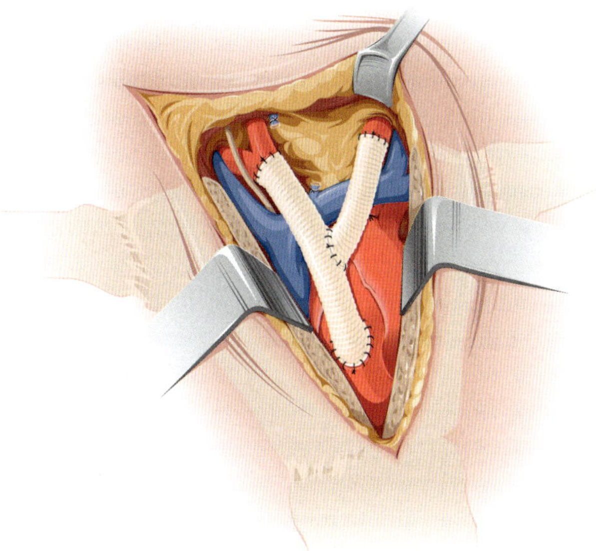

FIGURE 4.6. The most frequent arrangement: aorto-IA–Lt CCA bypass through an upper sternotomy.

as some have recommended. If a standard bifurcation graft were to be used, it would have a #16 trunk with limbs of 8 mm in diameter in order to match the diameter of the CCA. The slanted shape to which the proximal end of the #16 mm graft must be shaped to achieve a tangential anastomosis with the ascending aorta would result in a large perimeter anastomosis that requires a considerably larger opening in the aorta,

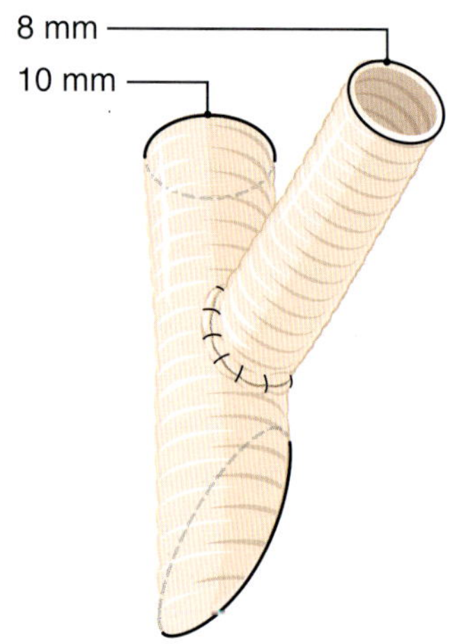

FIGURE 4.7. The enlarged perimeter of the slanted proximal anastomosis.

hence, a greater exclusion clamping of the ascending aorta. Furthermore, the bulk of the pressurized trunk of a #16 mm graft in the anterior mediastinum may actually either compress the brachiocephalic vein or be compressed itself by the sternum.

Another reason to prefer the #10/#8 configuration is better conditions for flow and more physical similarity with human geometry. From a mechanics point of view, the ideal area ratio for an arterial bifurcation is 1.16. The area ratio of a #10 tube with a #8 side branch is 1.64. In contrast a #16 × 8 commercial bifurcated graft has an area ratio of 4.61. This will result in a pressure drop at the bifurcation of the prosthesis and will cause a high percentage of wave reflection. I do not know if these disturbed flow circumstances have any impact on outcomes but I suspect they will not be better than those obtained with the smaller and more physiologic configuration of 10 + 8, described above.

If the distal anastomosis of either branch is to be made at the carotid bifurcation, the most efficient way is to divide the CCA 3 mm below the flow divider. If a concomitant endarterectomy is indicated a Type 2 eversion is done and the graft is anastomosed end-to-end to the bifurcation (Fig. 4.8). The stump of the IA is closed with a continuous 4-0 suture between pledgets.

CERVICAL BYPASSES

Most cervical bypass operations aim to revascularize the SA from the ipsilateral CCA or vice versa.[2] Less common are the CCA–contralateral CCA bypass and the SA to contralateral CCA or ICA bypass. All revascularizations across the midline are done using the retropharyngeal route described below.

Revascularization of the CCA from the ipsilateral SA is indicated in patients with a severe symptomatic lesion of the CCA origin. The best solution is to *transpose the CCA to the SA*. The CCA is dissected into the mediastinum from a neck incision to provide adequate length for its transposition to the SA. The latter is usually an easily achievable step. The site for implantation in the SA can be the second or third segment of the latter. If adequate length is available, I prefer to transpose the CCA into the third segment, between the lateral edge of the scalenus anticus and the anterior

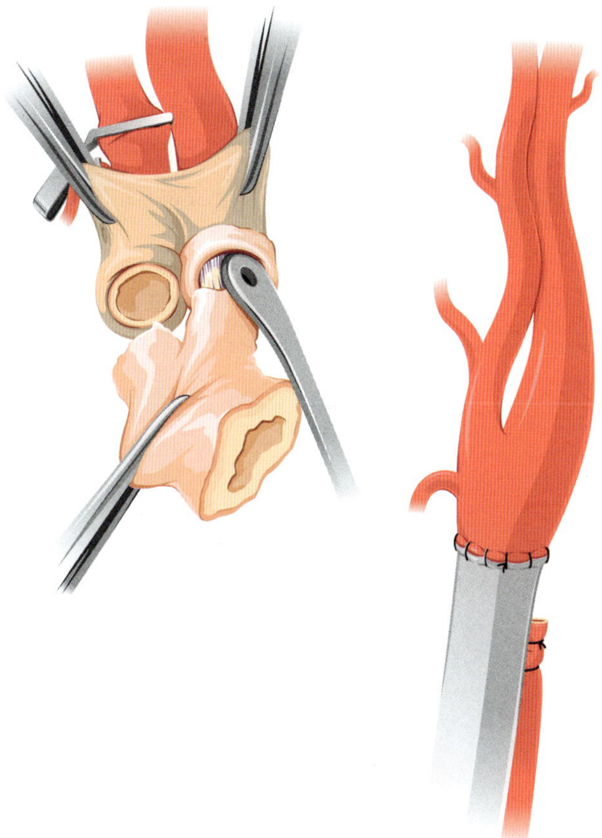

FIGURE 4.8. Distal anastomosis to the carotid bifurcation after eversion Type 2 endarterectomy of the latter.

cord of the brachial plexus. It is an easier access to the SA and avoids the full division of the anterior scalene muscle and the mobilization of the phrenic nerve.

Both transposition and bypasses are used to revascularize the SA from the CCA. The transposition is a good technique but requires a more demanding dissection, division of the scalenus anticus, and secure control of the proximal subclavian in the upper mediastinum from a neck incision. If the operation is done to correct embolization from a plaque located in the first segment of the SA, transposition is the better technique because it eliminates the possibility of any further embolization from the SA plaque, provides a simpler solution with a single anastomosis, and avoids prosthetic material. If the revascularization of the SA from the CCA is done to protect the former when covering its origin with an aortic endograft, the bypass is a more expedient technique.

Carotid–Subclavian Bypass

A short, 5 cm incision parallel to the clavicle provides access to both arteries involved in the bypass. Exposure of the SA is easier in its third segment at the gap between the anterior cord of the brachial plexus and the lateral edge of the scalenus anticus (Fig. 4.9). The first step is dissecting the periphery of the prescalene fat pad leaving attached the upper medial portion to be used as a hinge when reflecting the pad away

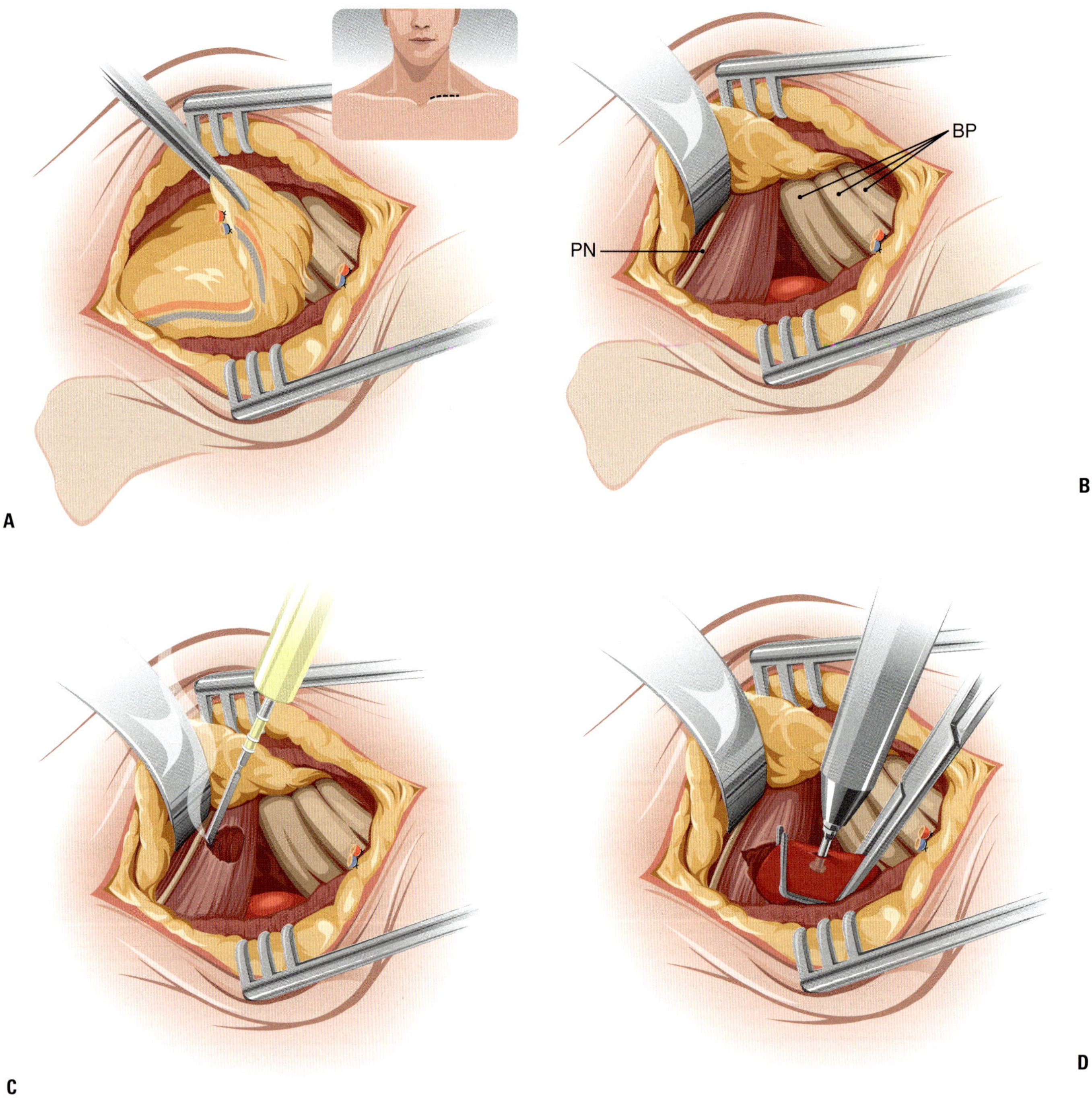

FIGURE 4.9. Steps in CCA–SA bypass. (**A**) Lifting the prescalene fat pad leaving it attached by a medial hinge. (**B**) Exposing the triangle formed by the SA, brachial plexus, and scalenus muscle. (**C**) Partial division of the lateral edge of the scalenus. (**D**) Punch arteriostomy of the SA. (**E**) Anastomosis to the SA. (**F**) Completed bypass.

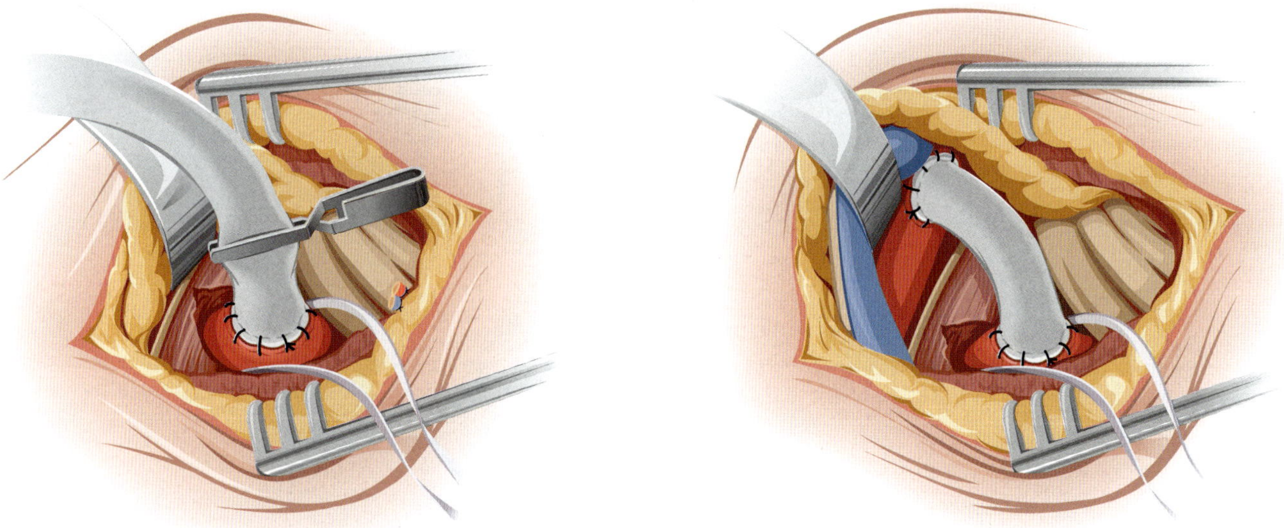

E F

FIGURE 4.9. (*continued*)

from the operative field. The homohyoid muscle is divided and the transverse scapular artery and vein are divided between ligatures. The SA is found in the inverted V formed by the anterior cord and the scalenus anticus. It may be necessary to divide the lateral half of the scalenus if the patient is corpulent and the exposure limited. In this case, prior to doing this, the phrenic nerve is located medial to where the lateral fibers of the scalenus will be divided. The third segment of the SA has one cervical ascending branch that does not have to be divided as it can be included in the clamp during the anastomosis.

The prosthetic is anastomosed to an arteriostomy in the SA made with a 5 mm aortic punch. The graft is passed under the jugular vein on to the lateral wall of the CCA to which it is anastomosed end to side.

BYPASS THROUGH THE RETROPHARYNGEAL SPACE ACROSS THE MIDLINE

The endotracheal tube is secured to the forehead in the midline to allow rotation of the neck during the operation as each side of it is dissected. The retropharyngeal space[ii] is accessed through the same incision used to expose the carotid bifurcation.

[ii] The idea for a retropharyngeal tunnel came during experiments done in dogs intended to define the relationship of axial flow velocity to the development of intima hyperplasia in a vein graft.[3] We intended to replace the CCA with a femoral vein graft and then bring the opposite carotid, across the neck, to be anastomosed to the mid-section of this vein graft, so that the only variant condition between the proximal and the distal half of the graft would be the flow velocity that would be approximately double in the proximal than in the distal half of the vein graft. After dissecting the carotid arteries on both sides of the trachea, it was obvious that by lifting the trachea and pharynx, we could easily bring the opposite carotid across the midline and reach the vein graft. The carotid arteries were only 3.5 cm apart in the prevertebral plane. Incidentally, this is the same plane followed by the rSA in a human.

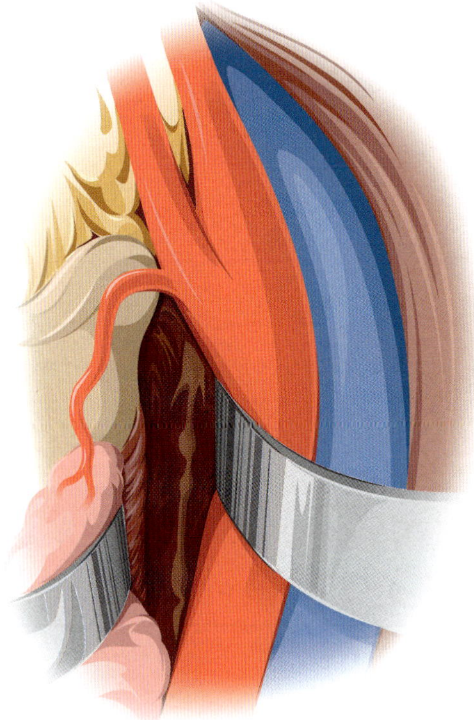

FIGURE 4.10. Approach to, and development of, a retrophyaryngeal tunnel.

Once the CCA is isolated (Fig. 4.10), the sympathetic chain is identified behind it.[3,4] The surgeon's finger goes over the sympathetic chain and is directed posteriorly and toward the midline till it slides over the lamina prevertebralis and palpates the anterior lips of the bodies of the cervical vertebrae. Once it has crossed the midline, the finger is slid up and down in front of two vertebral bodies to make room for the future graft in what was till then a virtual space. As this is done, the pharynx is displaced away from the vertebra by the dorsum of the exploring finger. If our intention is to do a SA–contralateral CCA bypass, the retropharyngeal space can be reached from the subclavian site by slidding the finger over the scalenus anticus and the longus colli until it reaches the unmistakable anterior surface of the vertebral bodies.

We follow the same procedure in both sides of the neck and leave a Penrose drain in the prevertebral tunnel that will help pass the graft from one side to the other. The distance between the two CCAs through the retropharyngeal tunnel is 5 cm. This distance, if the bypass is placed anterior to the trachea, doubles to 10 cm (Figs. 4.11 and 4.12).

The possibility that a prevertebral, prosthetic graft may interfere with pharyngeal function has been raised.[5] Postoperative endoscopy of the first six retropharyngeal bypasses I did failed to show any bulging of the graft in the posterior wall of the pharynx. Only 1 of the 47 patients that to date underwent retropharyngeal bypass had temporary swallowing difficulty. In this patient a swallowing test showed malfunction of the pharyngeal constrictor.[iii]

[iii] A likely explanation for the temporary swallowing deficit in this patient might have been excessively wide freeing of the posterior pharynx from its attachments to midline soft tissues, while making the tunnel, causing a paresis of the IX nerve.

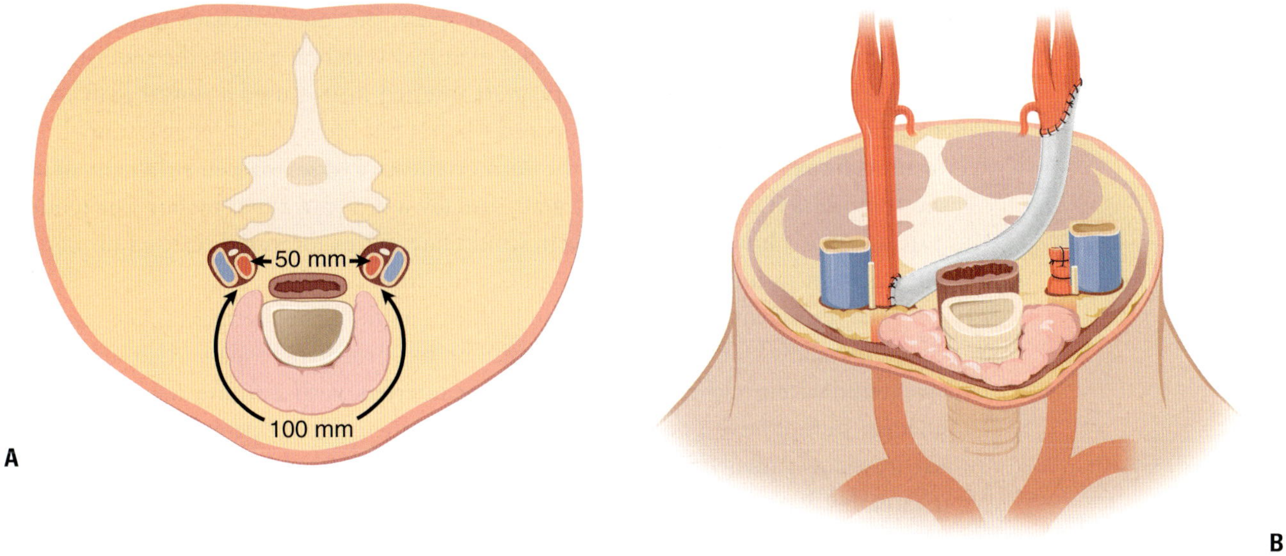

FIGURE 4.11. The retroesophageal route is one-half the length of the pretracheal route.

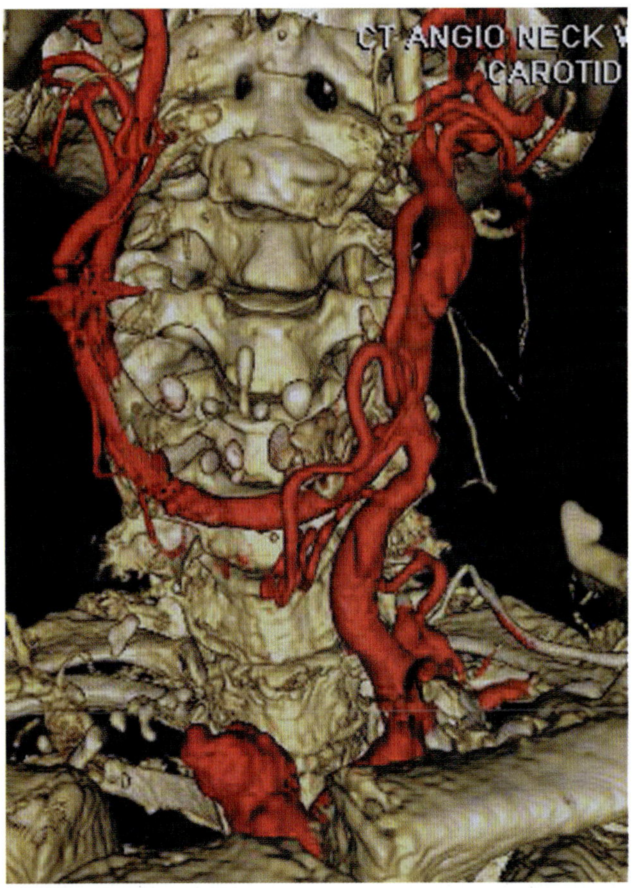

FIGURE 4.12. A carotid retropharyngeal bypass provides Rt carotid inflow in this patient whose only branch from the arch is a Lt CCA.

The retropharyngeal space is a virtual space, but once we have introduced the finger across it and developed this space over two vertebral bodies, the resulting tunnel does not compress the prosthetic graft inserted in it. I used a ringed graft in one patient who had had neck radiation and where I felt the retropharyngeal tunnel tight against the exploring finger with the head extended. I have not seen either any extrinsic compression of the prosthetic graft (usually a 7-8 mm tube) by bone or tendon. I do not know how a saphenous vein would fare in this location because I do not use the latter for reconstruction of the supraaortic trunks.

The retropharyngeal route is one-half the length of the pretracheal one and consequently allows for a shorter, and hence better, prosthetic bypass. Also, unlike the conventional pretracheal grafts, it does not interfere with a future tracheostomy or median sternotomy, a not uncommon event in the future of patients with advanced arthrosclerosis involving the supraaortic trunks. The retropharyngeal route is a simpler pathway to revascularize the contralateral side when a patient has only one patent branch arising from the arch (Fig. 4.13) if a sternotomy is to be avoided.

Bypass of a symptomatic lesion of the IA can be done through a cervical approach using the retropharyngeal route (Fig. 4.14). A short supraclavicular incision gives access to the third segment of the Lt SA. A right carotid incision with a posterior "boomerang" extension will expose the Rt CCA and the Rt SA. The retropharyngeal tunnel is developed first from the left side by sliding the finger over the scalenus anticus (and then the longus colli) till the anterior lips of the vertebral bodies are felt.

On the right side, the CCA is isolated medial to the IJV and dissected proximal to near its origin. If the operation is done to relieve an IA occlusion, rather than to treat an embolizing IA plaque, retrograde flow from the lower CCA will supply the

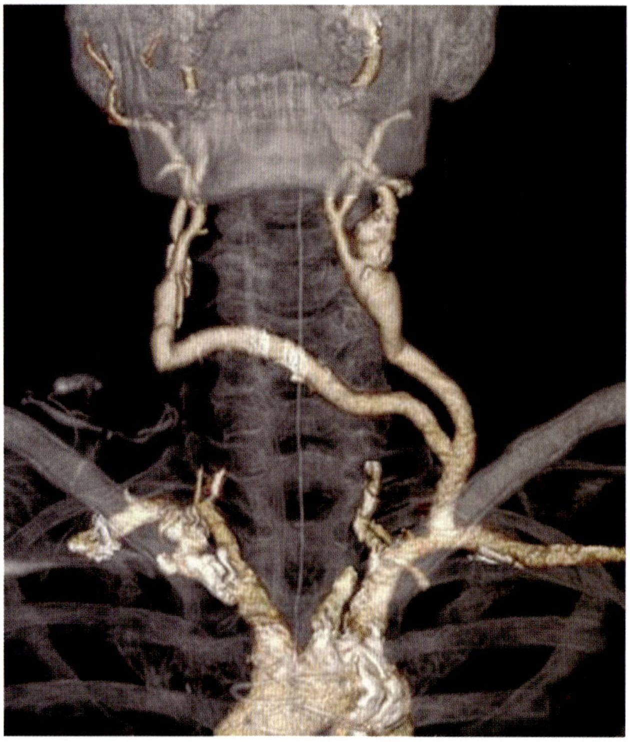

FIGURE 4.13. Bilateral carotid revascularization from the Lt SA.

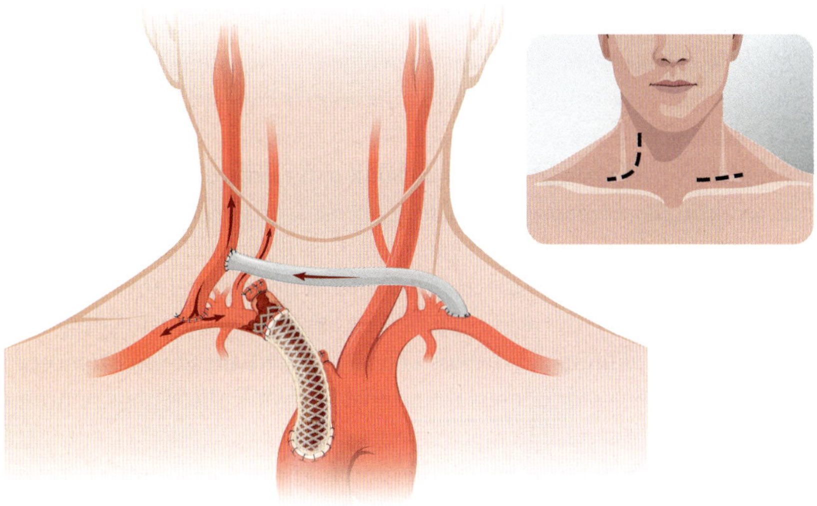

FIGURE 4.14. Schematic of a cervical approach to bypass a symptomatic occlusion of a previously stented IA in a patient who had two previous sternotomies for coronary and valvular disease.

SA and the VA. If the operation requires exclusion of the IA lesion (because of evidence of embolization from it) the Lt SA–Rt CCA bypass (usually 7 mm PTFE) is completed and open to distal flow. Next, the proximal Rt CCA is divided close to its origin and the now free proximal CCA is transposed under the IJV and over the vagus to the superior wall of the SA to which it is anastomosed end to side (Fig. 4.15).

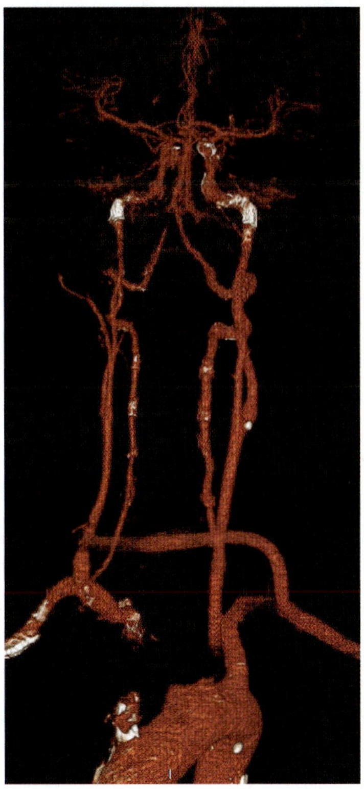

FIGURE 4.15. Retropharyngeal revascularization for a symptomatic IA occlusion.

PROBLEMS TO AVOID

A *tear of the brachiocephalic vein* can be avoided by opening the sternal retractor slowly and in small steps while monitoring the stretch imposed on the vein by inspection and palpation.

The application of a partial exclusion clamp to a calcified plaque in the ascending aorta can result in *local dissection*, *rupture of the wall*, or *distal embolization*. The preoperative CTA and direct inspection can identify problematic areas where clamping is to be avoided. If a torn wall is noted at the time of declamping after construction of the proximal anastomosis, the repair can best be handled by inducing deep hypothermic arrest with cardiopulmonary bypass. The #10 graft, already anastomosed to the ascending aorta, can be used to insert the arterial line while the venous return cannula is placed in the readily accessible superior vena cava.

When placing the drain in the mediastinum at the conclusion of the repair, a long clamp is advanced retrosternally to the subxyphoid drain exit. Unless the clamp is advanced parallel and close to the undivided lower sternum, it could *injure the right ventricle.*

A Lt VA that has a *low origin in the Lt SA* (3% incidence) presents a problem when trying to transpose the SA to the Lt CCA because the cervical approach does not permit to dissect and divide the SA close to its origin in the arch. In this case the VA is first transposed to the CCA before transposing the SA to an adjacent CCA site.

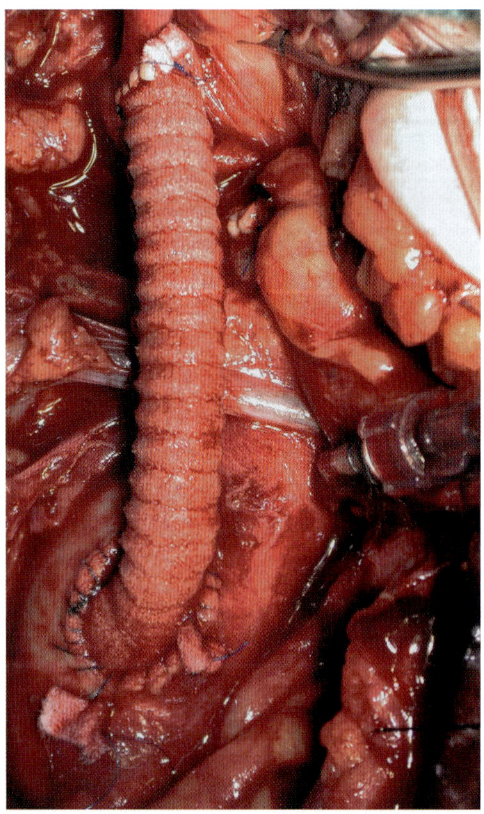

FIGURE 4.16. A short catheter inserted in the aortic arch provides accurate pressure monitoring when there is extensive atherosclerotic disease of the extremities.

During construction of an ascending aorta–IA bypass it is of utmost importance to have a reliable central blood pressure display, given that the surgeon is rendering the patient hypotensive and this may drastically decrease brain inflow. Patients with extensive disease of the SAT often have lesions in both SA and iliofemoral segments that may invalidate the pressure measurements recorded from a peripheral arterial line. In these patients a direct catheter inserted into the arch will provide easy and reliable monitoring (Fig. 4.16).

OPERATIVE RISK FOR SAT RECONSTRUCTIONS (1981 TO 2010)

	N	Stroke		Death	
		N	**%**	***N***	**%**
TT	146	9	6.0	7	4.0
CE	263	7	2.0	1	0.4

REFERENCES

1. Berguer R, Morasch MD, Kline RA. Transthoracic repair of innominate and common carotid artery disease: immediate and long-term outcome for 100 consecutive surgical reconstructions. *J Vasc Surg.* 1998;27:34–42.
2. Berguer R, Morasch MD, Kline RA, Kazmers A, Friedland MS. Cervical reconstruction of the supra-aortic trunks: a 16-year experience. *J Vasc Surg.* 1999;29:239–248.
3. Berguer R, Reddy D. Intimal hyperplasia. *Arch Surg.* 1980;115:332–335.
4. Berguer R. The short retropharyngeal route for arterial bypass across the neck. *Ann Vasc Surg.* 1986;1:127–129.
5. Berguer R. Revascularization by the retropharyngeal route for extensive disease of the extracranial arteries. *J Vasc Surg.* 1984;1994:217–215.

CHAPTER 5

Operations on the Internal Carotid Artery

INDICATIONS FOR CAROTID SURGERY

The general adoption of the single metric of percent stenosis to select patients for intervention or operation is regrettable. It allows the treatment of some lesions that could be left alone and discards intervention in others that should be operated. Currently, it is generally accepted that in the absence of conditions that would increase the surgical risk or decrease life expectancy, endarterectomy should be considered in asymptomatic patients who have an ICA plaque causing a 70% to 99% stenosis. And having placed too much importance in this arbitrary boundary (70%) for intervention has probably resulted in inappropriate management of symptomatic patients with lesions of less than 70% diameter stenosis (with the usual pathologic features: hypoechoic plaque, ulceration, etc.) and unnecessary operations in asymptomatic, benign lesions causing a narrowing greater than 70% diameter.

And then, there are lesions that although clinically asymptomatic they present with ipsilateral "silent" infarcts seen in the CT (hence "signomatic"). The reason some infarcts are clinically silent is that the impaction of embolic material took place in an area that has no obvious clinical representation. Silent infarcts, however, result in the same long-term brain deterioration that is seen in infarcts that presented with TIA or stroke. It makes sense to apply to these signomatic lesions the same criteria for intervention that we use for symptomatic ones. There are two categories of patients with carotid lesions in whom the percent stenosis range limit should not apply: patients with "silent infarcts"[1] because their plaques have already showed their embolic potential, and symptomatic patients (hemispheric/ocular TIA or stroke) who have a bifurcation plaque with the structural features (deep ulceration or surface thrombus) that cause embolization.

POSITIONING AND PROTECTIVE INTERVENTIONS

The patient is supine with a thin roll behind the shoulders and adequate support for the head so that at no time the latter is hyperextended or not fully supported. The head is turned away from the side of the operation. Before induction it is advisable to try the position of the neck in which the patient will be placed to detect the rare case where a patient cerebral perfusion depends on his VA supply and becomes symptomatic when the neck is turned and VA flow arrested.

The medication protocol for carotid endarterectomy includes the following: heparin 10,000 U IV, dextran 40, 100 mL push (plus 50 mL/h $\times$ 3), and dexametasone 10 mm IV.

As more patients are exposed to endovascular heparin from percutaneous diagnostics and interventions, the base dose of 10,000 U may not achieve the desired activated coagulation time of 300 seconds. If this is the case additional 5,000 U doses are given.

Dextran is a polysaccharide made of chains of glucose of different lengths and hence different molecular weights. Dextran 40, the one used in clinical medicine, is a low molecular weight dextran (40,000 Da) more easily excreted by the kidney than the heavier dextrans. Approximately 75% of dextran 40 is excreted within 24 hours of its administration. Dextran 40 increases the electronegativity of red blood cell and platelet membranes, decreasing their adhesiveness and platelet clump formation. The dose specified in this protocol has little risk of causing overload and cardiac failure. Anaphylaxis from dextran is rare and is even less common with low molecular weight dextrans.

In addition to using dextran IV at the time of heparinization, I use dextran topically to clear and wash the endarterectomy surfaces because once adsorbed onto the surface it will decrease platelet deposition on it when flow is resumed. Another advantage of using dextran to cleanse the endarterectomy surface is that it is a birefringent solution that, when the headlight is shown upon it, makes easy the identification of the small media debris that remains after the endarterectomy.

Dexamethasone given as a single 10 mg dose provides protection against an unknown allergy of the patient to X-ray dye or to dextran itself. But, more importantly, it decreases swelling secondary to brain ischemia. I am not aware of any downside of using a single 10 mg dose of dexamethasone during operations on the VA or CA.

In the 1970s much debate centered on whether or not a "shunt" should be used during carotid clamping, and whether there was a way of selecting those patients in whom the shunt would be necessary to avoid ischemia. There were futile attempts at trials and metaanalysis to sort out the significance of the use of a shunt in postoperative stroke amid the myriad variables involved in carotid operations.

I used a shunt routinely during the first 5 years of practice, then only in those patients with a contralateral occlusion and practically never in the last 15 years. During the time I used shunts I had the opportunity of observing some of the complications derived from the use of this presumably protective tool, such as intimal tears, short dissections, and atheromatous embolization from its proximal end "scooping" a grossly diseased CCA.

Those that advocate measuring the *ICA "back-pressure"* would insert a shunt when the back-pressure reading is <25 mmHg. With these criteria they end up inserting a shunt in 10% of patients. This is clearly an overuse since not using a shunt at all results in less than 1% of ischemic accidents in large personal series, including mine, and even in this fraction of 1% of patients, it is more likely that embolization from a technical flaw rather than low perfusion is the source of the infarction.

EEG monitoring complicates the operative setup and could only be of help if it could differentiate ischemia due to low perfusion rather than embolization. Actually, an embolus in the basal ganglia or occipital lobes will not be detected. A frontoparietal embolus, if detected, will surely stress the surgeon but its ischemic consequences will not reverse by inserting a shunt.

Doing the carotid endarterectomy under *regional anesthesia* and interrogating the patient periodically has also been used as the ultimate test for the need of a shunt. Again this results in an overestimation of the need for a shunt. In terms of cerebral blood flow one would expect a large decrease from 50 mL/100 g/min (normal) to 20 mL/100 g/min to cause unresponsiveness. But this level of relative ischemia, unless prolonged, is not damaging to brain cells and function will return when perfusion returns to normal levels.[i] Furthermore, if a deficit arises the probability of it being secondary to microembolization is still high and no improvement can be expected in such a case from the insertion of a shunt. A shunt may be the source of potential problems in exchange for avoiding a rare mechanism of intraoperative stroke: critical hemispheric decrease in blood flow.

HYPOTHERMIA IN "ARACHNIDS"[ii]

Most intraoperative brain infarctions are embolic, though some are the result of inadequate perfusion to a bed that has no adequate collateral supply. The longer the ischemic period, the more likely that neuronal death will occur. This situation may appear when operating on an isolated carotid that has no connection to the contralateral carotid (absent A_1 and pCom) or, more commonly, when a patient who has a single remaining vessel directly supplying the brain, hence an "arachnid" (Fig. 5.1),

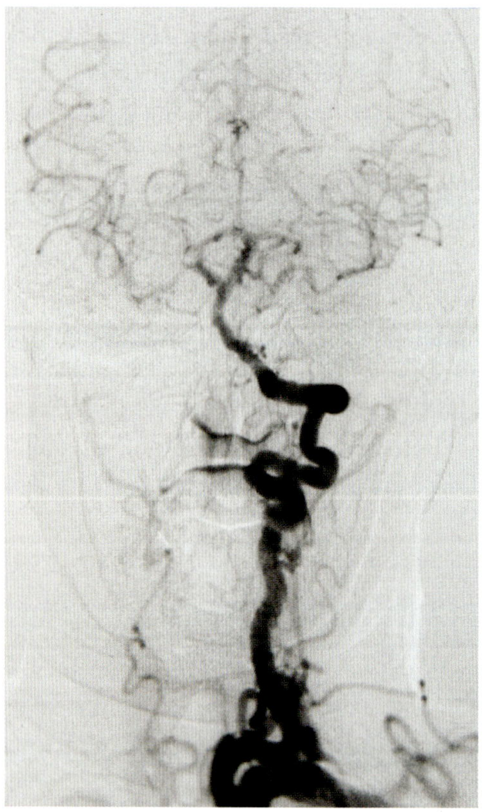

FIGURE 5.1. The Lt VA in this patient is the single blood supply to the brain.

[i] I was performing an endarterectomy under regional anesthesia (uncommon in my practice) in a patient with a small (about 3 mm) ICA. When the anesthesiologist informed me that the patient had become unresponsive 4 minutes after clamping I tried, unsuccessfully, to insert a shunt. I gave up fearing I would tear the artery and proceeded to complete the endarterectomy as expediently as possible. The patient woke up immediately after resumption of flow and experienced no neurological deficit.

[ii] A lax allusion to the vascular system of spiders that have a single contractile vessel that functions as a heart.

needs a reconstruction of this one vessel and there is no possibility of shunting. The rationale for using *moderate hypothermia* (33°C) when operating in these circumstances follows.

Brain damage caused by low flow or no flow is time dependent. A short arrest or severe decrease in flow, as we see in ventricular fibrillation or severe hypotension, does not result in neuronal death. Prolongation of the flow arrest impairs the blood–brain barrier, causes edema, suppresses cellular function (firing), and eventually damages cellular integrity. Damage will occur first in those tissues with the highest metabolic rate.

Hypothermia has a remarkable protective effect over the consequences of flow arrest. Different *levels* of hypothermia result in different protective effects. The *time span* between the ischemic insult and the state of hypothermia also determines the degree of protection achieved by the latter. Animal experiments have shown *that protection is maximal if the ischemic insults occur when the brain has already been cooled.* Conversely, the longer the delay between the ischemic insult and the cooling, the less protective effect the latter affords. If hypothermia is started beyond 2 hours after the ischemic insult, it has no protective effects.

With regard to the length of time that hypothermia needs to be maintained for neuroprotection the experimental evidence indicates that, when ischemia develops in an already cooled brain,[iii] the need for hypothermia may not be longer than 1 hour. This sequence of cooling prior to the start of ischemic injury fits well with the time sequence followed when using superficial hypothermia during operations on the ICA and VA: patients are cooled before clamping ischemia occurs.

There is solid experimental evidence that moderate hypothermia (33°C) results in a substantial decrease of cerebral metabolic rate (CMRO2) and a similar reduction in cerebral blood flow (CBF).[2] It also reduces the inflammatory response of the brain tissue to infarction.[3] It is estimated that *for each 1°C decrease in core temperature there will be reduction of* ±6% of the metabolic rate.

So, when the core temperature of a patient is lowered from 37°C to 33°C we should expect a 24% drop in metabolic needs. This will widen the time window under which the ischemic brain will be protected.

Mild and moderate hypothermia (35°C to 33°C) has been used in clinical studies to influence the outcome of an acute stroke. These studies used thermal blankets and jackets, bags of iced saline, and application of iced saline and alcohol to exposed skin. But these trials were marred by difficulties in dropping and maintaining the desired temperature, a problem compounded by heat generated by the shivering response in these awake patients.

In the surgical setting, the shivering response does not occur because cooling is not started until neuromuscular paralysis has been achieved during anesthesia. We use a cooling blanket and jacket as well as iced saline bags in the armpits and groins. Thin patients reach 33.5°C after approximately 30 minutes, but obese patients may require 1 hour or longer. When the temperature reaches 33.5°C cooling is stopped, the iced saline bags are removed, rewarming begins through the thermal blanket and jacket and the operating room ambient temperature is raised, regardless of the stage at which the surgeon is in the dissection. The core temperature (measured in

---

[iii] This is what experimentalists haplessly call "intraischemic hypothermia."

the bladder and in the larynx) will continue to drift down to 32.5°C to 33.0°C in the next 20 minutes. This is the time when the critical artery will be clamped and reconstructed. Rewarming will result in the temperature rising by about 2.0°C at the time of closure. Occasionally, after full reversal of heparin there may still be a slight increase in tissue oozing or suture hole bleeding because of remaining hypothermia. By the time the wound is closed, rewarming should continue and the patient is sent to recovery room on ventilator support not to be extubated until the core temperature reaches 36°C.

ACCESS TO THE CAROTID BIFURCATION

The incision, about 5 cm long, is oblique, almost transverse, curving around the angle of the jaw, 2 cm below it (Fig. 5.2). Once the platysma is divided and the external jugular vein (EJV) tied off, the dissection follows the anterior edge of the sternomastoid (SM) muscle. By lifting the proximal edges of the wound, the SM dissection is prolonged for another 4 to 5 cm below the edge of the wound so that later the SM can be retracted away from the jugular vein.

Rarely an unsuspected low bifurcation or a severely calcified CCA may require to expose the CCA lower for later clamping. To extend the incision inferiorly we follow the anterior line of the SM and divide the omohyoid muscle. The vagus tends to become anterior to the CCA as we dissect the latter towards the mediastinum. For this reason the dissection of the CCA begins in its anteromedial wall.

In the upper part of the incision we may encounter the auricular nerve. This nerve can be displaced upward by dividing the muscular roof of its tunnel (platysma) and mobilizing the nerve posteriorly.

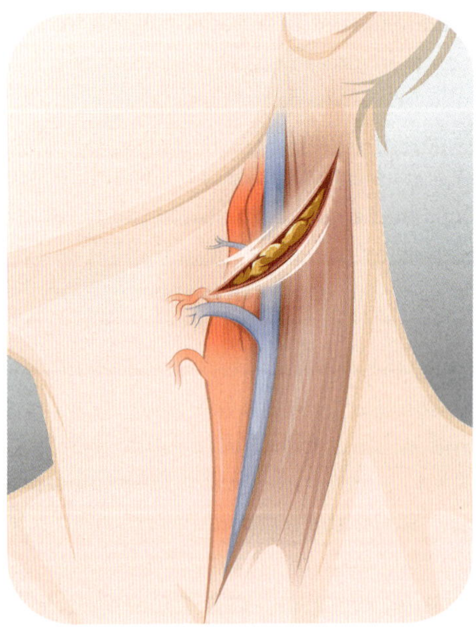

FIGURE 5.2. Incision to access the carotid bifurcation.

In individuals with a large parotid gland the lower tip of the superficial lobe is lifted from the SM and held inside the upper retractor. Distally, the tenddinous anterior edge of the SM is identified and the dissection follows on top of this tendon until the digastric muscle is met. The dissection of the internal jugular vein (IJV) starts at the bottom of the field and proceeds upward until the facial vein is identified and divided (Fig. 5.3). As the dissection continues on the anterior edge of the IJV, the next good-size vein that we encounter will be the one we call the "hypoglossal" vein because it usually covers the hypoglossal nerve (in a high bifurcation the facial vein may be the one covering the XII nerve). Before dividing this "hypoglossal" vein, we verify by that no underlying nerve is visible through the vein wall by tugging upward the right angle clamp and flattening the vein.

The CCA is isolated first bearing in mind the possibility that the vagus nerve may be anterior below the bifurcation. The vagus is dissected away from the CCA and this freeing of the nerve continues upward toward the top of the incision. Next the external carotid artery (ECA) and ICA are isolated. The superior thyroid artery is temporarily occluded with a hemoclip. During dissection of the superior thyroid artery or when placing the hemoclip, one should avoid damaging the flimsy external branch of the superior laryngeal nerve which frequently can be seen resting on the 1st cm of the superior thyroid artery (Fig. 5.4) (see Section "The Carotid Artery" in Chapter 1).

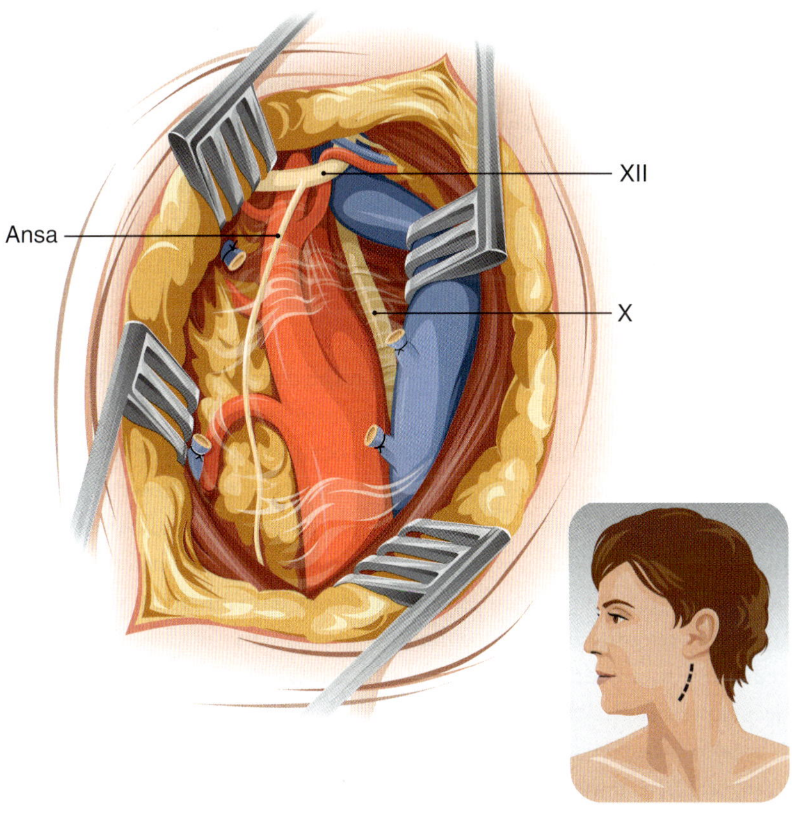

FIGURE 5.3. Posterior retraction of the IJV exposes the bifurcation.

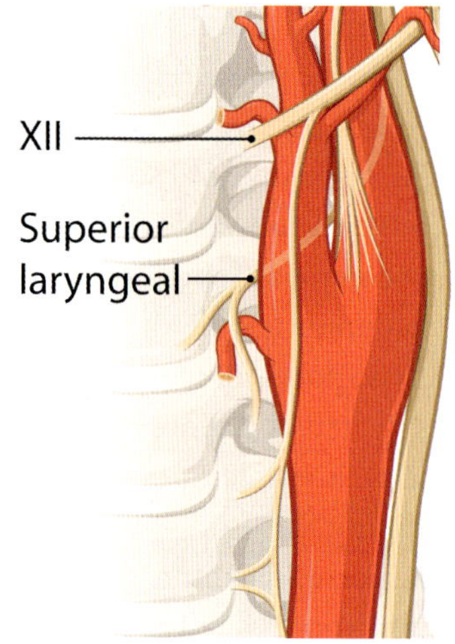

FIGURE 5.4. Relationship of the external branch of the superior laryngeal nerve to the superior thyroid artery.

The ICA is dissected distally for as long as needed till a healthy gray-blue color in the entire perimeter of the artery indicates that there is no plaque at this level.

PROXIMAL EXTENSION

If the bifurcation is unexpectedly low or the quality of the distal CCA is not adequate for clamping (because of extensive calcification), the *exposure needs to be prolonged proximally*. If undermining the lower flap of the incision does not suffice, the skin incision is extended vertically.

DISTAL EXTENSION

When the bifurcation is unusually high or when the distal end of the carotid plaque is above the level of the hypoglossal nerve, the *exposure may need to be extended distally.* The digastric muscle is first divided. Next the occipital artery (or its sternomastoid branch as may be the case) is divided as it loops over and tents down the hypoglossal nerve. Once the XII nerve is free it can be displaced anteriorly allowing more exposure of the ICA. If further length of distal ICA is required, the artery is approached above the XII. In this case it is of essence to avoid damaging the glossopharyngeal nerve as it crosses over the ICA. Once the hypoglossal nerve is mobilized and the ICA is dissected above it, an additional 2 cm of this artery can be freed.

If the plaque reaches the level of the hypoglossal nerve or higher, the best way to handle it is to *transpose the ICA in front of the nerve* (Fig. 5.5). For this, the ICA is divided at its origin, as if for a Type 1 eversion, and then pulled under and then over the hypoglossal nerve leaving the latter posterior to the artery. This allows straight traction of the ICA to free additional length distally. In this case, when reanastomosing the ICA, after the eversion endarterectomy, the artery is left anterior to the hypoglossal nerve.

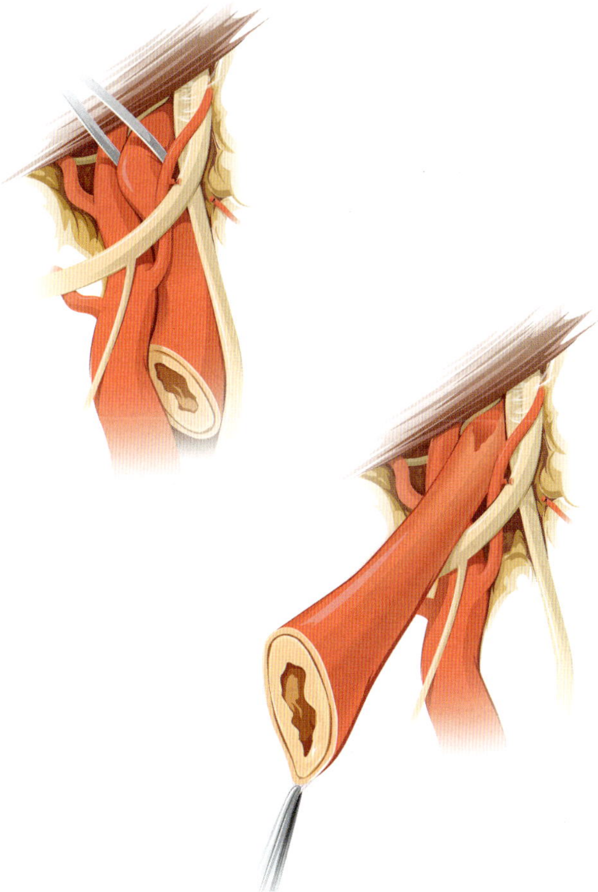

FIGURE 5.5. After severing its origin, transposition of the ICA in front of the XII nerve permits further distal dissection of the former.

RETROJUGULAR ACCESS TO THE INTERNAL CAROTID ARTERY AT C2

The retrojugular[iv] approach permits exposing the ICA up to the C1–C2 level. If control of the ICA is needed above C1, then the anterior infratemporal approach (see below) should be chosen. The incision for the retrojugular approach is the same as that described for standard exposure of the carotid bifurcation (Fig. 5.6). The difference here is that the dissection starts behind the IJV between it and the SM (Fig. 5.5). The accessory spinal nerve is identified 2½ fingerbreadths below the mastoid tip. Once the nerve is isolated and looped to protect it, the ICA is exposed by retracting the IJV and the vagus nerve anteriorly (Fig. 5.7).

[iv] This is an approach to the high cervical ICA whose usefulness became obvious during distal VA reconstructions. When the V3 segment of the VA is exposed after flipping the jugular vein and vagus nerve anteriorly, the middle segment of the cervical ICA is unobstructed by the hypoglossal nerve.

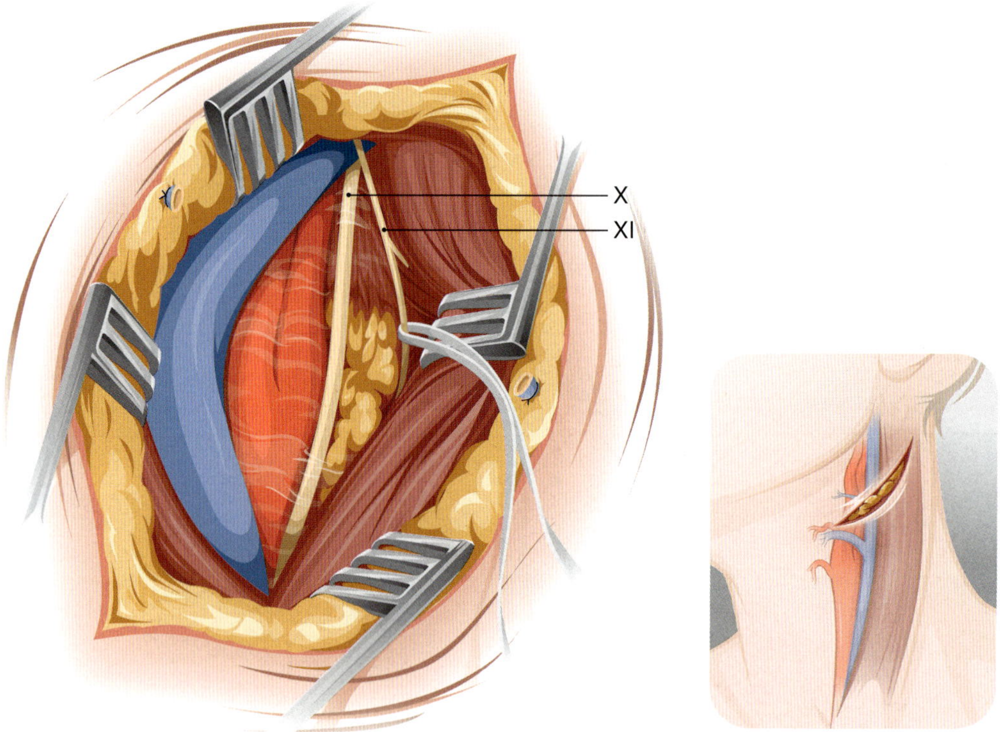

FIGURE 5.6. Retrojugular approach to the midcervical ICA.

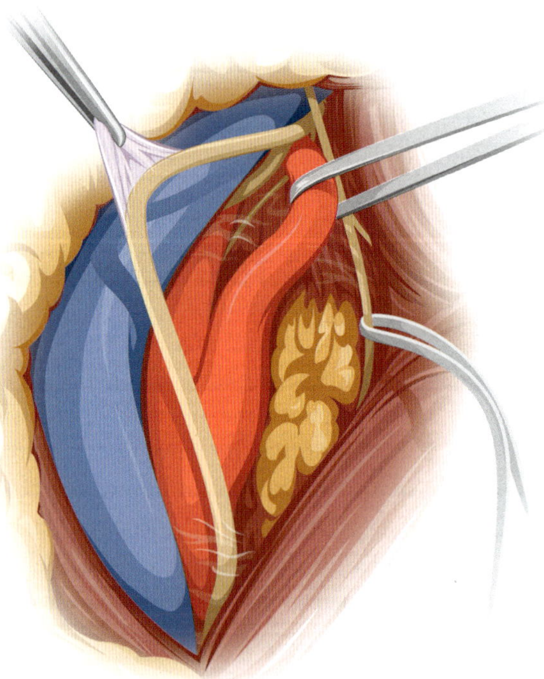

FIGURE 5.7. The ICA is isolated after flipping the IJV and the X nerve anteriorly.

In this approach, the carotid bifurcation is exposed without the need to divide the facial vein. Above the bulb the ICA can be dissected without the encumbrance of the hypoglossal nerve that has been displaced anteromedially with the vagus and the IJV. The carotid can be dissected up to the takeoff (from the vagus) of the superior laryngeal nerve that crosses behind the ICA at the level of C2. Behind the exposed ICA, at the level of C2, lies the superior cervical ganglion.

DISTAL EXTENSION TO C1 (MANDIBULAR SUBLUXATION)

If the extent of the needed exposure had been anticipated to reach within 1½ cm below the temporal bone, we would have done a *mandibular subluxation* prior to the skin incision after the patient has been intubated naso-tracheally (Fig. 5.8). The subluxation is unilateral and should produce a 10 to 12 mm of underbite on the subluxated side. The mandible is maintained in place either with arch bars or with a wire loop through the anterior nasal spine and around the mandible.

The occipital artery and the digastric muscle are divided. The dissection proceeds above the XII nerve identifying the glossopharyngeal nerve that crosses over the ICA (Fig. 5.9). The IX nerve needs to be protected from traction or thermal injury that can result in disabling dysphagia. Just above the IX nerve the fingerpad of the surgeon rotated cranially palpates the sharp, bony styloid process. The latter is exposed with a key elevator and its distal two-thirds as well as the attached stylohyoid ligament are removed with a rongeur. The facial nerve is posterior to the styloid process and could suffer thermal injury if electrocautery is used at this level.

Distal control of the ICA is best achieved with a short balloon catheter (Fig. 5.10). The edges of the distal ICA are held with two sutures to facilitate reinserting a balloon in case of accidental pulling of the catheter or puncture of the balloon during the anastomosis.

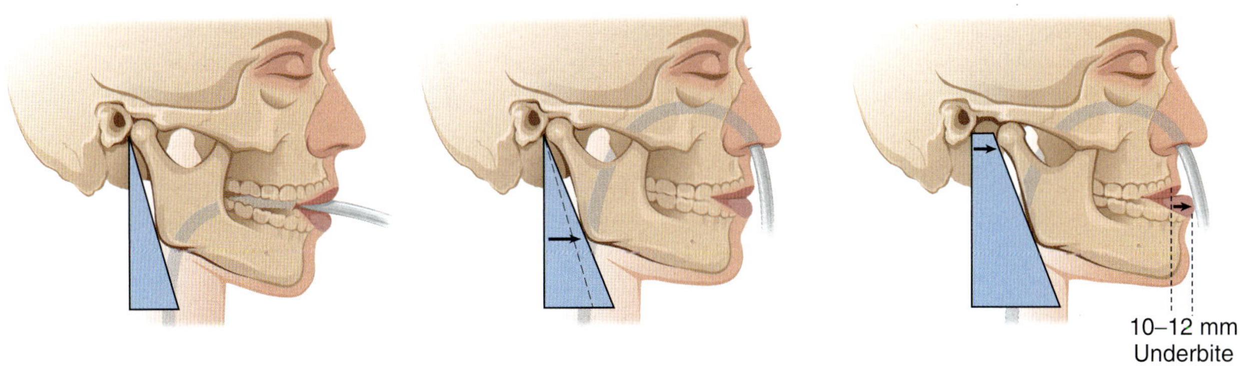

FIGURE 5.8. The relative contribution of endotracheal intubation (mid-frame) and subluxation (right frame) to the exposure of the distal ICA.

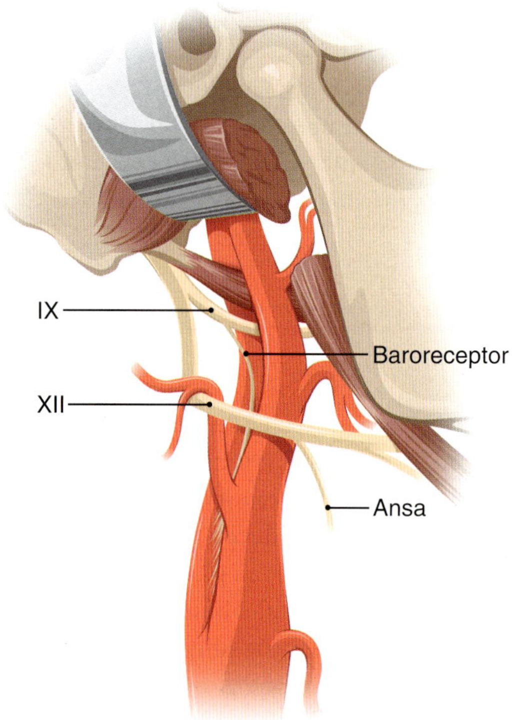

FIGURE 5.9. Schematic of the anatomy involved if the distal ICA is exposed.

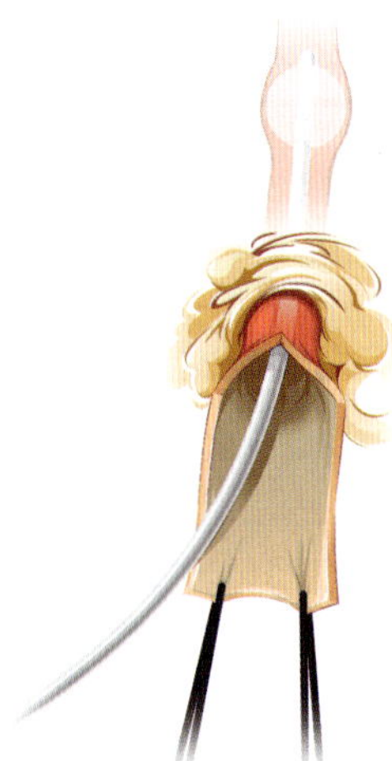

FIGURE 5.10. Distal control of the infratemporal ICA with a balloon catheter.

POSTERIOR APPROACH TO THE INFRATEMPORAL INTERNAL CAROTID ARTERY

The infratemporal ICA can also be approached posteriorly. The upper cervical ICA, when approached from the posterior neck, lies in a trough whose bony sides are the cervical spine medially and the jaw laterally (Fig. 5.11). In this approach the mandible does not cover or obstruct access to the high cervical ICA. From the posterior

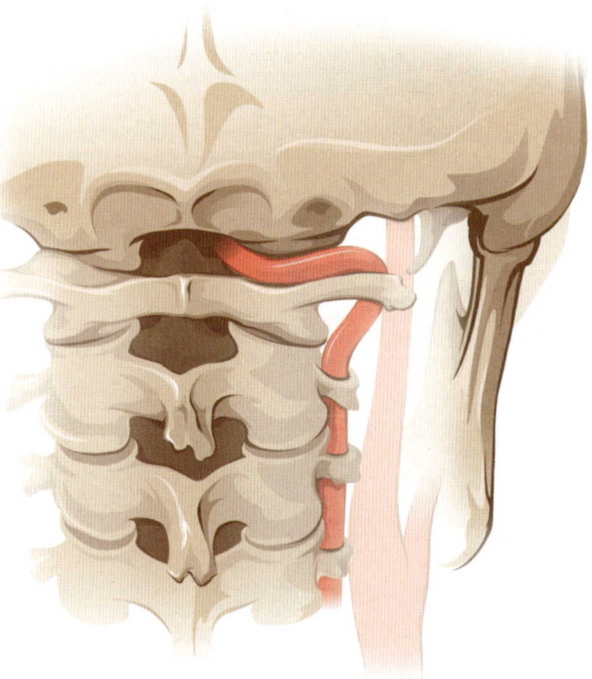

FIGURE 5.11. Relationships of the distal ICA and VA to bone structures from a posterior approach.

approach,[v] the infratemporal ICA is covered by the X, XI, and XII cranial nerves that need to be isolated and gently retracted away to mobilize the underlying carotid at this level (Fig. 5.12).

STANDARD CAROTID ENDARTERECTOMY

The dissection starts in the CCA and proceeds cranially isolating the ECA and ICA. Once adequate anticoagulation is achieved and the systolic blood pressure has been stable at 135 to 140 mmHg, the ECA and ICA are occluded with micro-clamps. A pediatric ductus clamp occludes the CCA after having chosen by palpation a safe site for it (Fig. 5.13A). The arteriotomy that follows starts in the CCA and is carried over the ICA as far as necessary to visualize the end of the plaque once the artery is opened.

The arteriotomy is started in the CCA and veers slightly toward the posterolateral aspect as it crosses the bulb and extends along the ICA to a level that will permit visualization of the distal end of the plaque. If plans for a *shunt* have been made this is the time to place it.[vi] The endarterectomy begins in the thickest portion of the

---

[v] This posterior approach became feasible while isolating the suboccipital VA above C1 (see Section "Suboccipital Approach to the Vertebral Artery at C0–C1" in Chapter 6), to treat a patient with a symptomatic vertebral dissected up to C1 that would not respond to anticoagulant therapy. The operation was to be a vein bypass to the suboccipital VA and it made sense to try to isolate the distal ICA for proximal inflow through the same operative field (Fig. 5.12).

[vi] In the few cases (3%) where I use a shunt I prefer the T-type with a side branch that permits to aspirate any debris that may have been collected by the proximal end of the shunt when it is advanced into the proximal CCA. The shunt is set in place with two saline-filled balloons. I use an additional Javid clamp proximally and gentle traction of a Pott's tied silastic loop to secure both balloons in place.

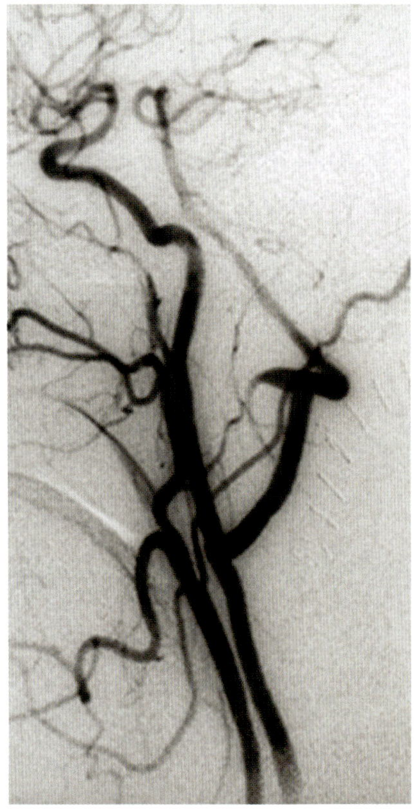

FIGURE 5.12. A bypass to the suboccipital VA takes origin in the infratemporal ICA. Both arteries were approached posteriorly. The carotid bifurcation is below the frame of the picture.

plaque where it is easier to encounter the proper plane. The lifting of the plaque begins in the CCA (Fig. 5.13B). If there is no proximal feathering of the plaque, as is often the case, a right angle clamp placed around the plaque permits cutting the latter flush. The step created by cutting the plaque proximally (Fig. 5.13C) will be later smoothed by folding over it the adjacent endarterectomized surface (Fig. 5.13D). Next, the ECA component of the plaque is freed. At this level one should try transitioning the endarterectomy plane to a more superficial layer so that it may feather off the ECA easier.

If the ECA plaque is concentric it will seldom have a feathering point and it is best to cut it sharply against the wall. If, on the other hand, the plaque is eccentric and the perimeter of the ECA does not show underlying plaque, the endarterectomy is continued and can be expected to feather well.

Attention is now turned to the ICA. As the surgeon approaches *the distal* end of the plaque a transition must be made from the outer to the inner lamina (Fig. 5.14). This will provide a fine feathering point and avoid the possibility of a flap.

The surface where the endarterectomy has been done is now debrided of bits of media that run transversally like the hoops of a barrel. These remaining bits are best seen by irrigating the surface with dextran 40 which, being birefringent, improves their visualization when the headlight shines on them.

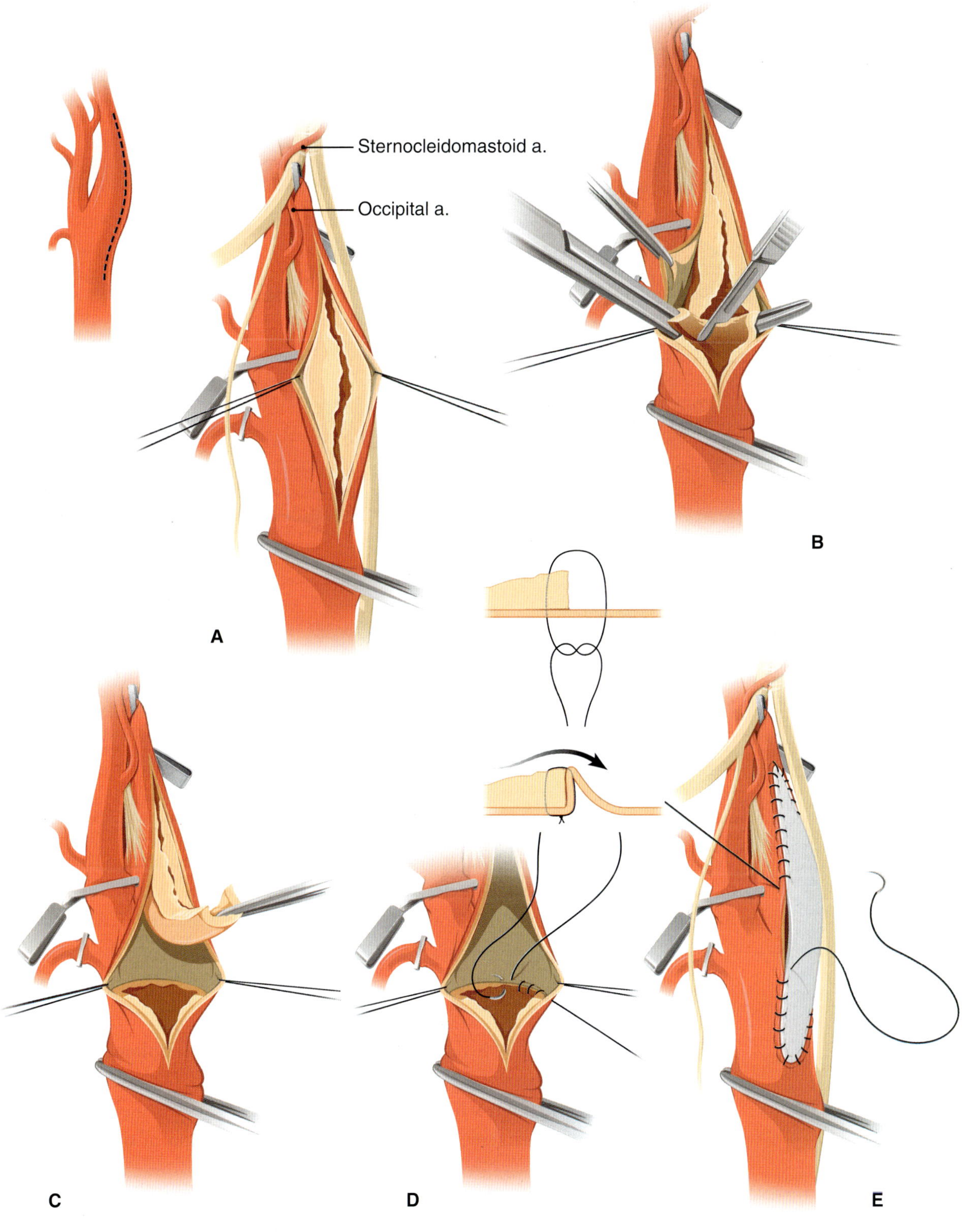

FIGURE 5.13. (**A**) The carotid bifurcation dissected and clamped. (**B**) Endarteretomy begins at the CCA. (**C**, **D**) The sharp step created by the transection of the plaque in the CCA is covered with the adjacent endarterectomized wall.

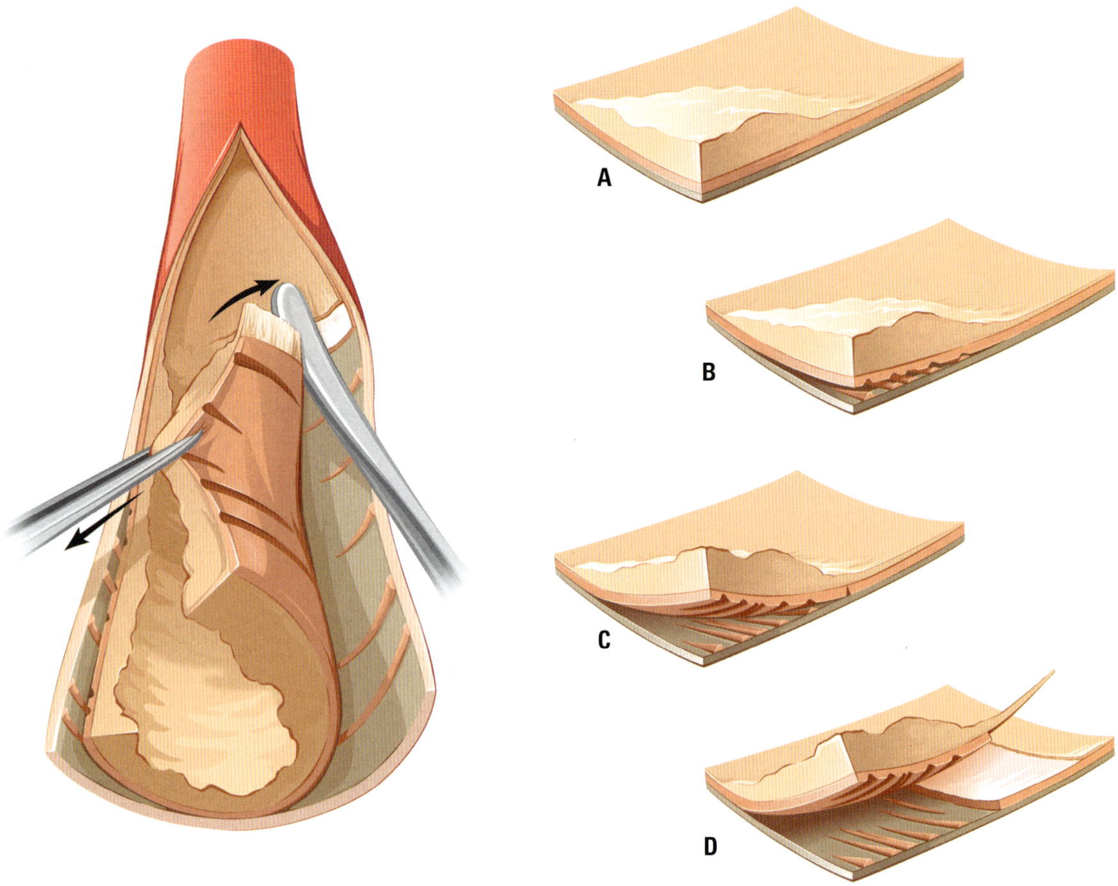

FIGURE 5.14. The endarterectomy plane becomes more superficial (internal elastic) near the end-point to avoid creating a distal flap. A combination of rotation and counter pressure with the endarterectomy spatula allows termination of the endarterectomy at the right plane.

With the exception of the few cases where the diameters of the bulb and ICA are particularly large, the arteriotomy is closed with a patch sewn with 6-0 suture (Fig. 5.13E). After appropriate back bleeding flow is resumed into the ECA and the ICA.

EVERSION ENDARTERECTOMY[vii]

In *Type I* eversion the ICA is detached from its origin with an oblique cut. In this technique the carotid baroreceptor nerves have to be divided. The ICA is stretched longitudinally and the point where its apex reaches in the CCA is used to mark the proximal limit of the enlargement of the orifice of the ICA. A cut of similar length is

[vii] The idea of an eversion endarterectomy happened during construction of the distal anastomosis of ascending aorta to carotid bifurcation bypasses. Often the carotid bifurcation was involved by atheroma and, once the distal CCA was divided in a slanted way, the plaque was removed by everting the bulb and the distal end of the graft was sewn as an end-to-end junction. It was obvious that the same thing could be accomplished by everting the bifurcation and then reanastomosing it. I started doing eversions for primary CEA in two manners: Type 1, amputating the ICA from its origin, and Type 2, transecting the distal CCA below the flow divider. While preparing a presentation of my experience with the first 100 eversion CEA,[4] I came upon a report by Etheredge,[5] who in 1970 had described the Type 2 eversion technique.

made in the heel of the opening of the detached ICA (Fig. 5.16A,B) which matches the opening in the CCA. If the ICA plaque continues into the CCA, as is nearly always the case, the distal CCA is endarterectomized first. The appropriate plane is

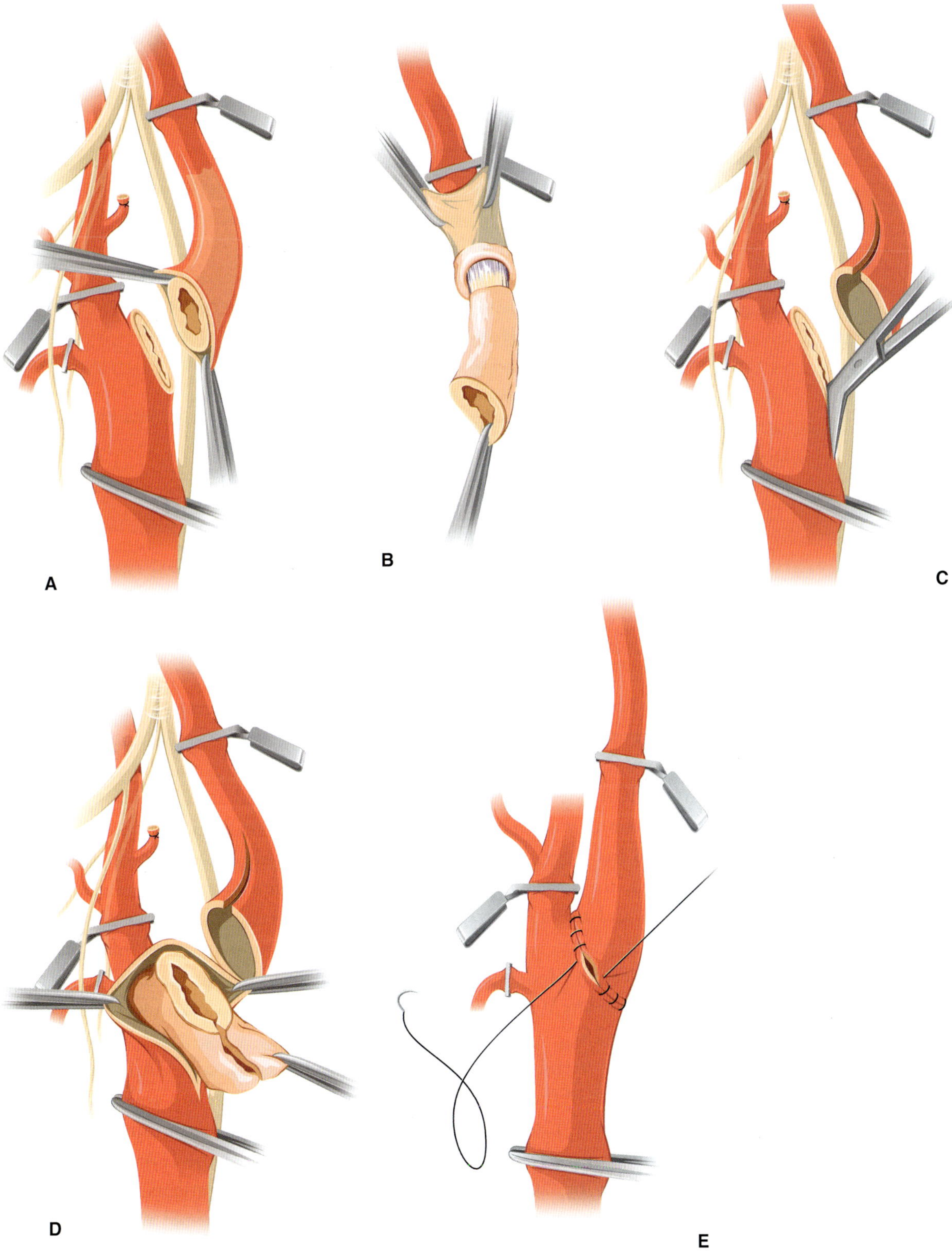

FIGURE 5.15. Steps for eversion endarterectomy Type I.

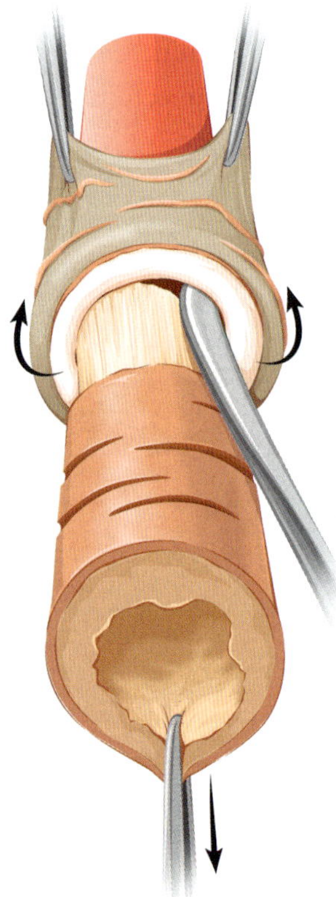

FIGURE 5.16. As the eversion endarterectomy progresses a "white crown" appears signaling the transition of the eversion endarterectomy plane to a more superficial level.

entered in both edges. A right angle clamp is passed underneath and the plaque is divided as proximally as feasible, flush with the right angle clamp. The plaque is then dissected from the origin of the ECA.

In the ICA, the endarterectomy plane is developed around its free end placing light downward traction on the plaque while an assistant provides countertraction of the free edges of the ICA (Fig. 5.16). As the distal end of the plaque is approached, the thin membrane of intima opposite to the tongue of the plaque tears open and the *white crown* of the internal elastic membrane appears as the thinned out plaque separates. The point of detachment of the plaque must be directly observed. Media debris is removed as described for the standard endarterectomy above. The ICA is reanastomosed to its widened origin with 6-0 polypropylene (Fig. 5.15E).

For a *Type II* endarterectomy (Fig. 5.17A–C) the distal CCA is divided 7 mm below the crutch of the bifurcation. The choice between Type 1 and 2 is determined by the proximal or distal extension of the bifurcation plaque. A plaque extending distally into the midcervical carotid is best managed with a Type 1. A plaque extending proximally into the CCA is best handled with a Type 2. Patients with a redundant ICA will be better managed with a Type 1 eversion combined with shortening of the ICA (Fig. 5.18). Occasionally, an ICA with inflammatory changes may, after a

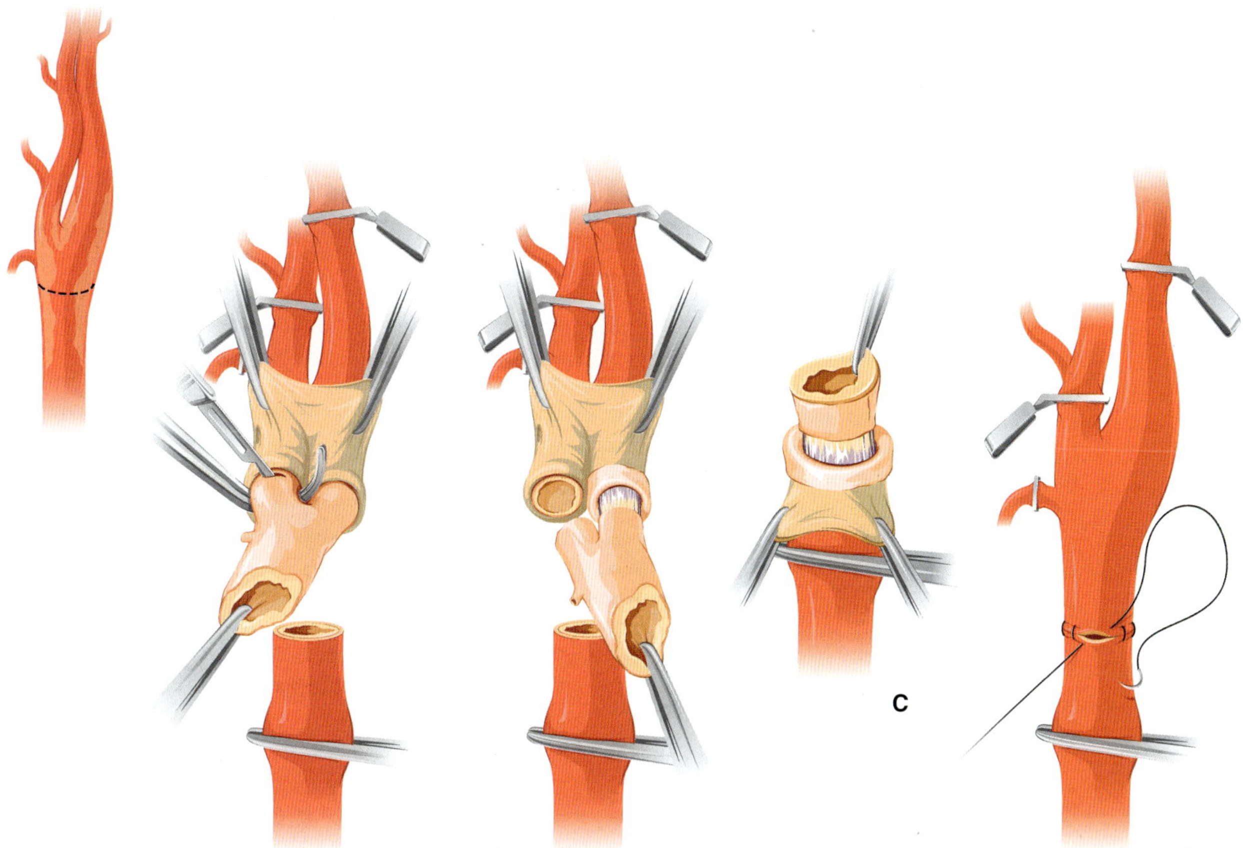

FIGURE 5.17. Eversion endarterectomy Type 2. (**A**) Distal "pantaloon" eversion with (**B**) the ICA freed last. (**C**) Eversion of the CCA and (**D**) Reanastomosis.

Type 1 eversion, appear to be of insufficient length to reanastomose it to the orifice in the CCA. If there is a question about tension in the suture line, the opening in the CCA may be extended through the ECA (Fig. 5.19).

TECHNICAL ERRORS

A *proximal clamp applied on a severely diseased* CCA may result in an operative stroke from embolization. Palpation of the CCA allows the surgeon to choose the best site for cross clamping. An extensively calcified CCA may need to be occluded with an intravascular balloon.

In Type 2 eversion, dividing the CCA too close to the flow divider will result in *a distal double channel* that will complicate the closure of the arteriotomy. One should bear in mind that the flow divider extends for about 5 mm below the external crutch of the bifurcation.

During eversion, the end of the plaque must be kept in open view. Detaching the plaque from beyond the point where it is visible may result in a *distal flap*. If the

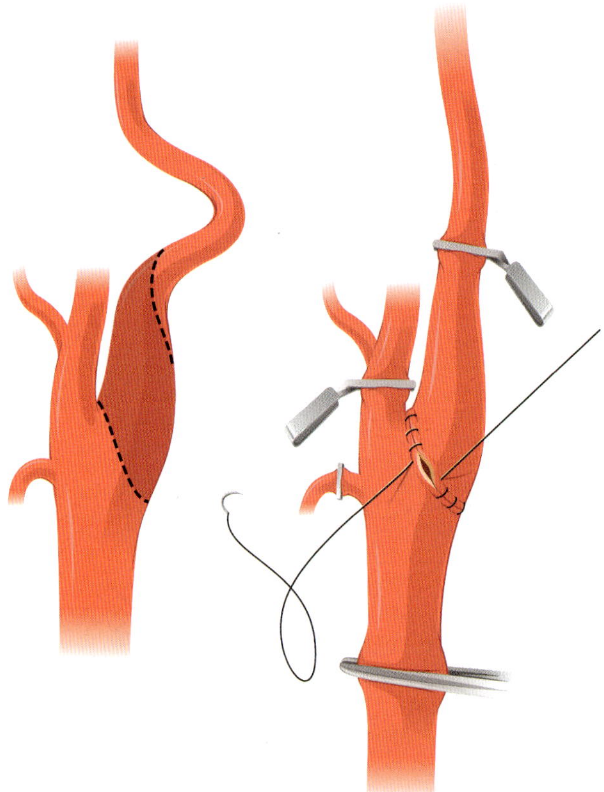

FIGURE 5.18. A redundant ICA is best handled by a Type 1 eversion.

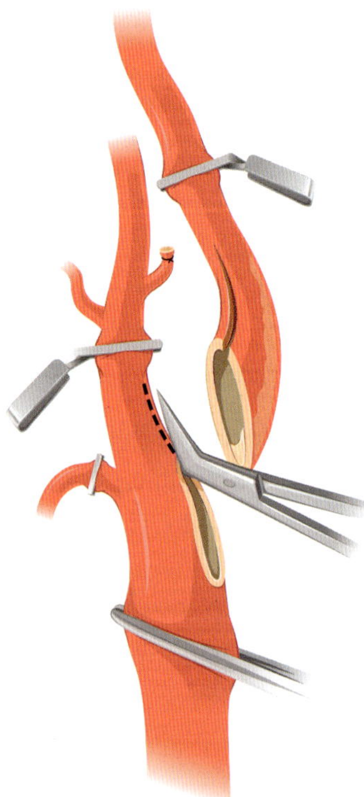

FIGURE 5.19. If, after a Type I eversion the ICA is under tension for its anastomosis to the CCA, the arteriotomy of the latter may be prolonged into the ECA.

surgeon does not routinely do completion arteriography, it is unlikely that this flap will be seen in an intraoperative duplex.

If a *plaque breaks and detaches before its feathering off point* is reached, the ICA will need to be reeverted to complete the endarterectomy. To accomplish this, a short #2 balloon catheter is advanced to the level of the upper occluding micro-clamp. Once the balloon is inflated, traction on the catheter coupled with the countertraction of the edges of the ICA will bring the remaining plaque into view and facilitate its controlled removal.

Atheromas with a high end-point often require dissecting higher than usual the postbulbar ICA. When doing so, one needs to exert traction on the artery while freeing its adventitia from the surrounding tissue. The intraoperative arteriogram will show an area of *spasm of the ICA* as a series of ring-like constrictions, similar to the mild lesions of FMD. These areas of spasm can be relaxed instantly by periadventitial infiltration of nitroprusside solution through a 27-gauge needle.

COMMON CAROTID ARTERY–INTERNAL CAROTID ARTERY BYPASS

It is not unusual that a carotid reoperation done for intima hyperplasia will develop a second recurrence, the restenosis appearing this time after a shorter interval from the operation that preceded it. In my experience with CCA–ICA bypass done for recurrent disease, PTFE thin wall grafts had a surprisingly better long-term outcome than autogenous saphenous vein grafts. The reason a 6 mm prosthetic tube functions so much better in this location than in the femoropopliteal area must be their high flow rate from lower peripheral resistance and absence of distal disease in the ICA.

In the treatment of recurrent disease, the advantage of the CCA–ICA bypass over patching (with or without endarterectomy) is that it minimizes redissection of the bifurcation and hence the possibility of injury to the X and XII nerves. The dissection for a CCA-ICA bypass starts proximal to the level of the previous operation in previously undissected CCA. Distally, the ICA is isolated above or below the XII nerve. The ICA is transected and the stump of the proximal ICA is suture ligated so that perfusion will continue through the ECA while the distal anastomosis is done. The latter is an oblique end-to-end junction that may be below or above the level of the XII nerve depending on where the ICA was divided. In the latter case, the bypass will lay anterior to the XII nerve. The bypass (a 6 mm thin wall PTFE) is then brought into proximity of the newly dissected proximal CCA and it is anastomosed end-to-side to it.

On a rare occasion, a surgeon may need to do a CCA–ICA bypass for recurrent disease in a patient who has occlusions of the contralateral ICA and both VAs. In this situation one may choose the protection of a shunt. The arrangement illustrated in Fig. 5.20 is a solution for achieving this that incurs in minimal ischemia time. The proximal end of the shunt is inserted first and secured with a sleeve tourniquet. The ICA is then divided above a miniclamp occluder and its distal end is cannulated with the distal end of the shunt. Once the shunt is secured distally by the inflated balloon, flow is resumed and the CCA is clamped above the proximal insertion site of the shunt. With the ECA clamped, a venous or prosthetic bypass can now be constructed between the segments bypassed by the shunt.

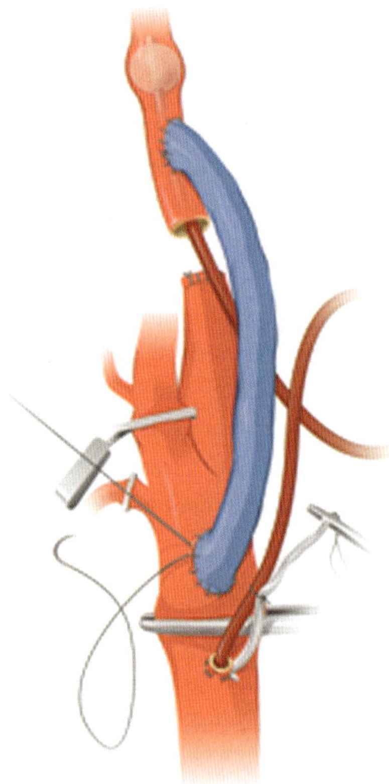

FIGURE 5.20. Placement of shunt before a bypass in patients with n other direct supply to the brain.

CAROTID REPLACEMENT DURING RESECTION FOR NECK CANCER

In patients with recurrent head and neck cancer the tumor often involves some component of the carotid bifurcation. It is not possible to determine if a recurrence adjacent to the artery is infiltrating its wall and any attempt to mobilize the artery away from the tumor is bound to leave residual tumor in the arterial wall or result in arterial injury. The potential cure for these patients is a resection *en bloc* of the tumor and adjacent vascular and neural structures. Ligation of the ICA in these circumstances carries a 30% risk of stroke. The stroke can be immediate, from uncompensated acute ischemia, or be delayed up to 3 days, from extension of the ICA thrombus into the MCA and ACA. This unacceptable risk can be avoided by reconstructing the carotid at the time of resection. Unfortunately, these operations for recurrent neck malignancy are likely to be contaminated by tracheal secretions, failure of skin flaps, or the development of a salivary fistula. If the ICA is replaced with a synthetic prosthesis, it is likely that the latter will become infected; a saphenous vein graft may also blow out if infected.[viii]

The question is then what material to use as carotid replacement. Encouraged by the short-term resistance to failure of arterial homografts in septic fields prompted me to use femoral autografts[6] to replace the carotid bifurcation in recurrent cases of squamous cancer of the neck.

[viii] I have seen two infected vein grafts rupture their wall after a carotid reconstruction for recurrent head and neck cancer.

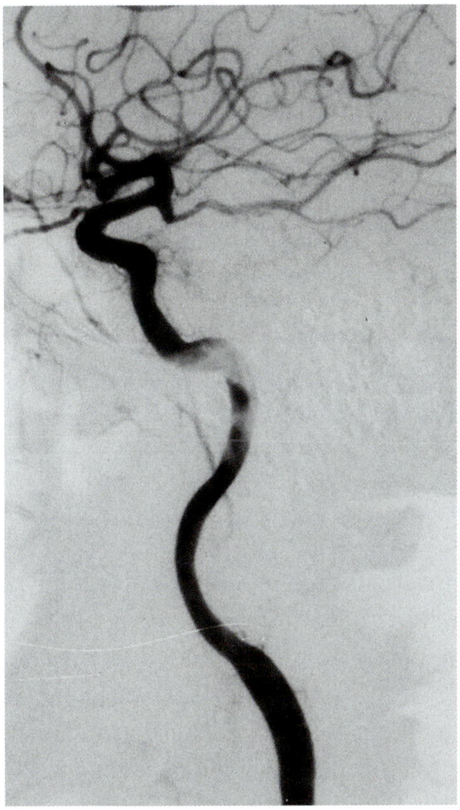

FIGURE 5.21. Replacement of the carotid bifurcation with a CCA–ICA autograft of superficial femoral artery.

The patients are US scanned preoperatively to ascertain the status of their superficial femoral arteries. If there is a segment of good quality, it will serve as an autografts for the resected carotid segment. The operation is planned with two separate surgical fields and instruments, assuming the head and neck field is, or will become, contaminated. In the separate sterile field, a segment of superficial femoral artery is removed and replaced with a PTFE graft. The graft is passed to the head and neck field to make an interposition graft between the CCA and ICA and the thigh wound is closed. The superficial femoral artery has a caliber conveniently between those of the CCA and ICA (Fig. 5.21). In our series of autograft carotid replacement in patients with advanced head and neck cancer,[6] 43% of patients developed wound infection or fistulization, but no graft thrombosed or ruptured.

REMOVING A FAILED STENT

Reconstruction of a previously stented ICA is best accomplished by dividing the origin of the ICA, in a manner similar to an eversion Type 1, with knife and then wire-cutting scissors. The proximal half of the stent lodged in the CCA is usually easy to remove by traction although irregular bits of tore intima will have to be cleared after dextran irrigation and illumination of the lumen of the CCA. Proximal control is best obtained with a temporary occluding balloon until a satisfactory surface is achieved. At this point a conventional clamp may be placed in the CCA.

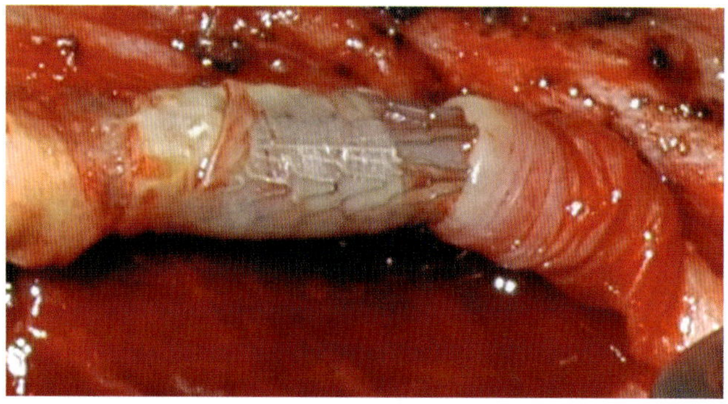

FIGURE 5.22. A stent and the tissue and compacted plaque that surrounds it are removed by eversion endarterectomy.

The distal part of the stent is removed by everting the ICA to a level beyond the distal end of the stent. The compacted atherosclerotic intima of the ICA generally remains attached to the stent (Fig. 5.22) so that the conventional eversion endarterectomy plane is followed. Any intimal flaps that may remain in the wall are trimmed under direct vision. The ICA is reimplanted into its origin, as is done for a Type 1 eversion endarterectomy. If the quality of the remaining wall of the ICA is in doubt, a CCA–ICA bypass with PTFE is performed.

RESECTION OF CAROTID BODY TUMORS

The reported experience with surgical resection of CBT carries the cogent message that the larger the tumor the greater is the risk of neurologic injury. A number of publications have reported the routine use of preoperative embolization to facilitate surgical excision and to decrease the operative blood loss. Preoperative embolization carries the risk of accidental embolization and stroke. The presumed advantage of decreasing bleeding during the operation is a weak argument given that primary surgical excision of a CBT does not require a blood transfusion.

Other authors have recommended excising the tumor with the ECA that bears the blood supply to the former or even resecting the entire carotid bifurcation and replacing the ICA with a vein graft. Any techniques that involve resection of the carotid bulb or the ECA complicate the simple excision of the tumor and add the risks inherent to clamping and manipulating the carotid bifurcation. A case can be made for discontinuing these extraneous procedures that increase the complexity, cost, and morbidity of these operations without having shown any demonstrable usefulness.

My practice is to resect the tumor using extensively a fine bipolar cautery for the control of the vessels on the surface of the tumor that have the appearance of small arteriovenous malformation channels. The ICA is freed from the tumor (Fig. 5.23). Both edges of the freed CBT open like a bivalve to expose the bifurcation and the supply of the tumor originating from the ECA. Generally, the last step in the resection of the tumor is freeing it from its attachment to higher ECA branches including the ascending pharyngeal artery (Fig. 5.24).

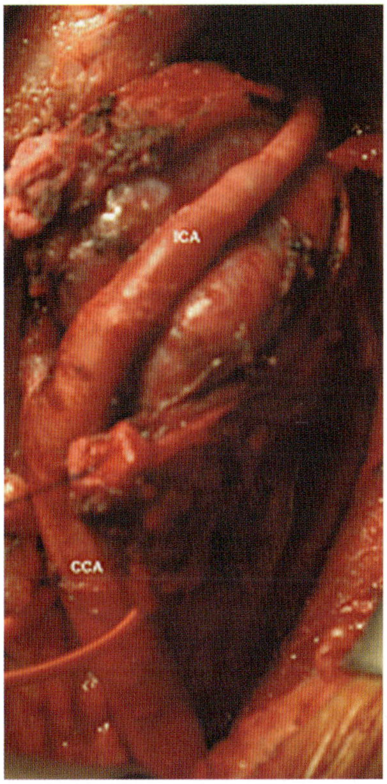

FIGURE 5.23. The ICA is freed between the anterior and posterior lobes of the CBT. The tumor, held by pledgeted sutures, is still attached to branches of the ECA.

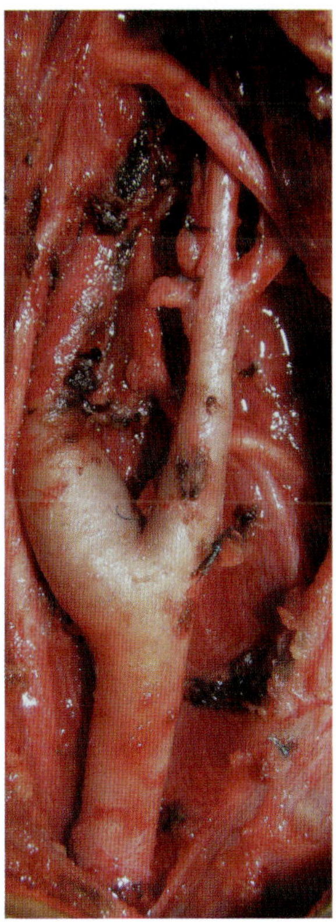

FIGURE 5.24. Carotid bifurcation after resection of a CBT. The superior laryngeal nerve is seen behind the empty bifurcation.

In as much as the size of the tumor correlates closely with the incidence of neurologic injury, when confronted with bilateral tumors it seems sensible to operate on the smaller, and hence less likely to result in neurologic injury, first, so that the second and larger tumor will not expose the patient to the possibility of bilateral cranial nerve palsy.

RESECTION OF CAROTID ANEURYSMS

Autogenous vein grafts used to repair *ICA aneurysms* have been reported to dilate, stenose, or kink.[ix] In Moreau's paper,[7] a savvy review of the extensive experience of Thevenet, 32% of the aneurysms were atherosclerotic and 21% were secondary to FMD (dysplastic). Seventy-four percent of patients presented with symptoms. They presented with a mass in the neck in 10% and into the pharynx in 5%. Most of the atherosclerotic aneurysms were located in the proximal ICA and involved the bulb. The aneurysms secondary to FMD were located in the mid or distal cervical ICA (Fig. 5.25). It is likely that the proximity of the ICA to the transverse process of C1 determines the high incidence of dysplastic aneurysms at this location: trauma of the ICA against the transverse process of C1 may result in a false aneurysm.

Suture line or patch failure will also result in an aneurysm (Fig. 5.26) and this is more likely to occur in an artery weakened by fibrodysplastic changes. Dysplastic aneurysms are also seen in patients with Ehler-Danlos (Figs. 5.27 and 5.28). Following

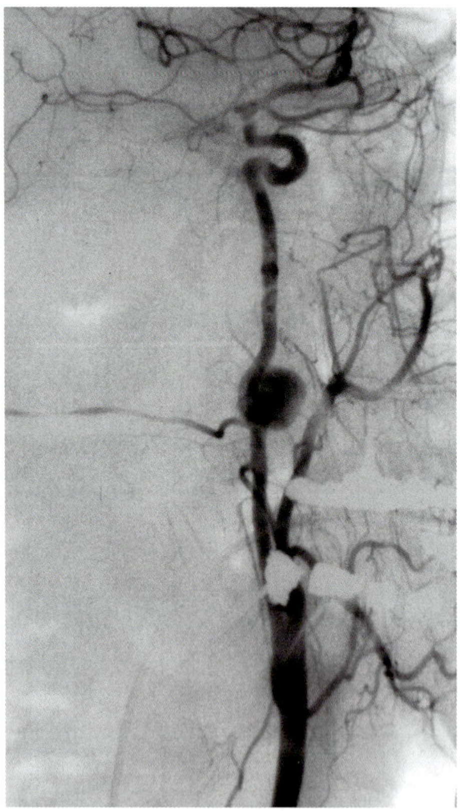

FIGURE 5.25. A dysplastic aneurysm in the mid-third of the cervical ICA.

[ix] I have seen the failure of a vein graft used to repair an ICA aneurysm in three patients with connective tissue disorders.

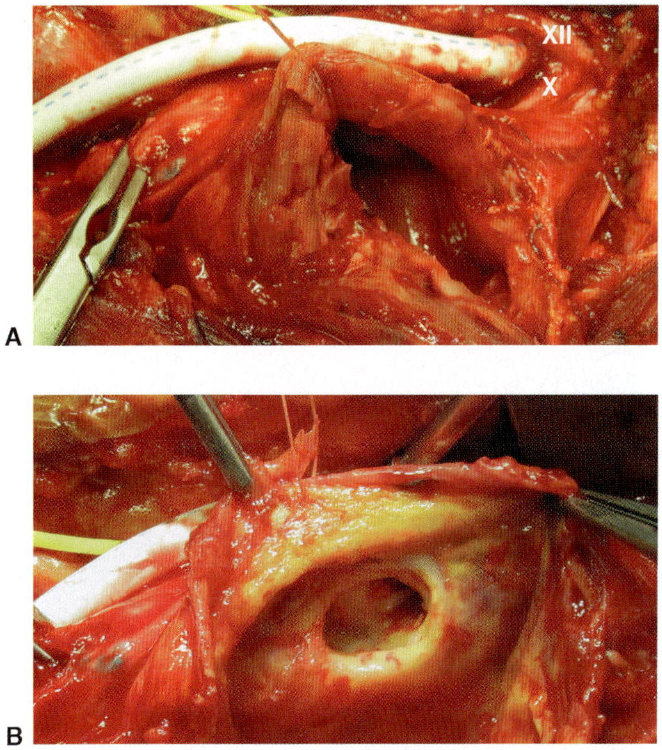

FIGURE 5.26. A false aneurysm (**A**) secondary to a failure of the suture line of a previous endarterectomy has been excluded by a bypass (CCA–ICA PTFE graft). (**B**) The defect in the previous suture line viewed from inside the aneurysmal sac.

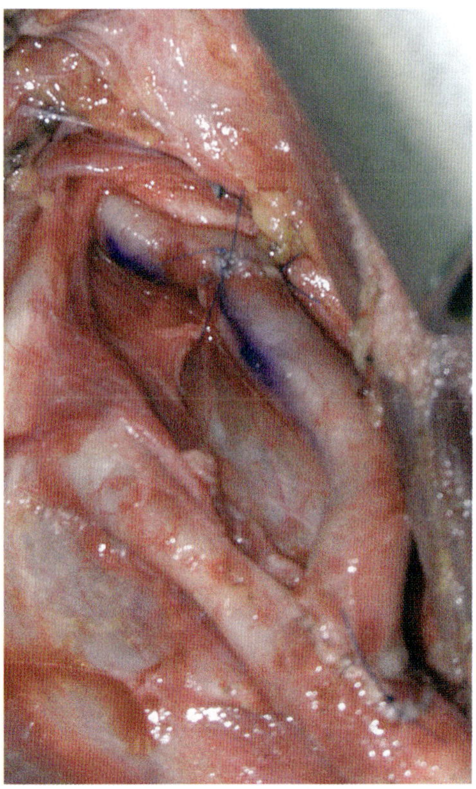

FIGURE 5.27. A vein graft replaces a dysplastic aneurysm of the ICA.

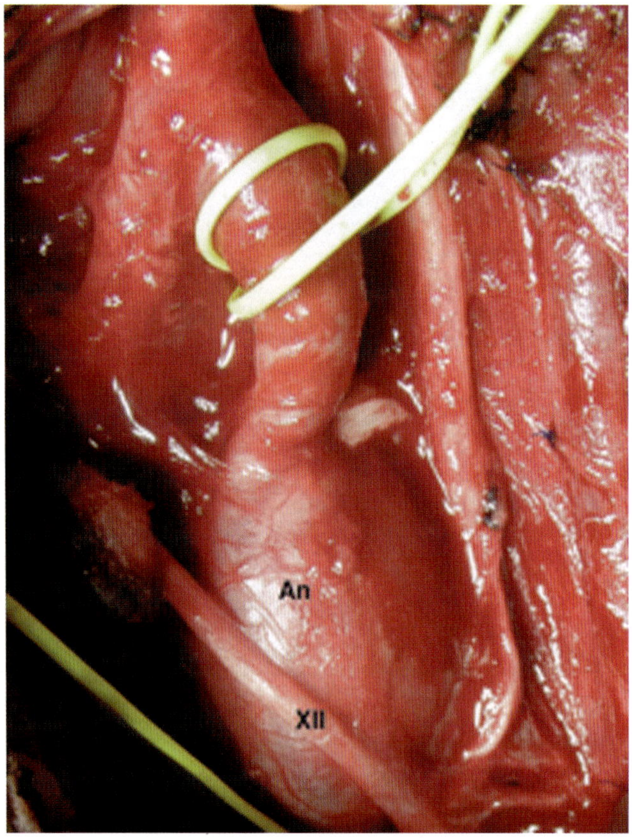

FIGURE 5.28. ICA aneurysm (An) above the XII nerve in a 20-year-old man with Ehler-Danlos.

resection of carotid aneurysm the incidence of cranial palsy (temporary or permanent) ranges from 22% to 44%.[7–9]

In cases with high aneurysms distal control is obtained with temporary intraoperative endovascular balloon occlusion. Ligation of the ICA to obtain thrombosis of the aneurysm is not an option for primary treatment as it is associated with a mortality of 20% to 40%.[10,11]

The preferred manner of obtaining vascular control of large ICA aneurysms is by proximal clamping, emptying the thrombus from the sac while allowing some back flow from the ICA and then inserting an occluding balloon into the ICA from inside the aneurysm to obtain distal control.[12] The distal anastomosis is made from inside the sac, as we do in abdominal aortic aneurysms, to avoid damage to cranial nerves that may occur during the external dissection of the distal neck of the aneurysm.

In aneurysms secondary to ICA dissection, the preoperative CTA will show if the false channel continues above the distal neck of the aneurysm. If a dissected wall is found at the level at which the graft will be anastomosed, the false lumen will need to be obliterated by apposition of both layers within the suture line. But this maneuver may not succeed to seal the distal dissection and the repair may be compromised or thrombosed by a false lumen pressurized by our incomplete seal of the anastomotic line or by another intimal tear beyond our anastomosis and not accessible from the surgical field.

NERVE INJURIES

Injury to the vagus nerve can be avoided by locating it as soon as the anterior edge of the IJV is freed from the CCA. Below the bifurcation the X nerve may drift its position toward the anterior surface of the CCA and could be injured when extending proximally the exposure of the latter.

The most common maneuver to result in *hypoglossal nerve injury* during exposure to the bifurcation is tying and transecting an anterior branch of the IJV that overlies and hides the XII nerve. This vein could be the facial (in high-lying bifurcations) or a vein entering the IJV above the facial (the "hypoglossal" vein). Because we do not know which vein may be covering the XII, all the veins draining into the IJV are hooked with a right angle clamp before their ligature. As the vein walls collapse over the jaws of the clamp an underlying XII nerve will be seen through the collapsed thin vein walls. The reports on hypoglossal injury rightly stress that nearly all the inadvertent injuries occur in the low-lying hypoglossal nerve in individuals with high carotid bifurcations.

The *glossopharyngeal nerve* is at risk whenever the ICA is dissected above the XII. The IX nerve is thinner than the XII nerve and may be injured when the surgeon liberates the ICA from it.

The *accessory spinal nerve (XI)* has a predictable location (2.5 fingerbreadths below the mastoid, under the anterior edge of the SM) but can be injured if, for some reason, the surgeon frees the posterior, rather the anterior, edge of the IJV when exposing the carotid bifurcation.

The *external branch of the superior laryngeal nerve* may be injured during isolation of the superior thyroid artery (see Section "Cranial Nerves and Sympathetics in the Carotid Bifurcation Field" in Chapter 1).

Parotid lifting neuropathy. See Section "Review of Technical Failures" in Chapter 6.

Palsy of the *marginal mandibular branch of the facial nerve* is a not infrequent consequence of an upper retractor pressuring this nerve against the edge of the mandible. Although in rare cases the trauma to the nerve may result in permanent asymmetry of the lips, function usually returns within 6 weeks.

MANAGEMENT OF COMPLICATIONS AFTER CAROTID SURGERY

The most frequent etiology for a *postoperative hematoma* developing in the recovery room is venous bleeding, often from a failed ligature of the facial vein. Clumsy extubation with straining and coughing is usually responsible for dislodging the ligature.

If the patient shows a *neurological deficit as anesthesia is being reversed* in the operating room, the patient has probably embolized during the operation. A less likely reason is a critical drop in blood flow during the operation. If the completion arteriogram had shown a flap or any other technical flaw that had been dismissed, the surgical field is reopened and the abnormality is corrected.

Otherwise the patient is placed on acute stroke protocol. In these patients that wake up from anesthesia with a central deficit an emergency non-contrast CT is often suggested to rule out a hemorrhagic infarction. This would be an extraordinary rare finding that I have never observed. Efforts should rather be directed to begin acute stroke therapy immediately.

A special case of paresis noted during anesthesia reversal is the patient who has had a previous stroke has recovered and presents now for an endarterectomy of the ICA supplying the previously infarcted hemisphere. The side previously infarcted will "wake up" from anesthesia later (15 to 20 minutes) than the contralateral intact hemisphere.

A *neurologic deficit* that develops in the recovery room, *20 to 60 minutes after the patient has awaken intact from anesthesia*, is caused by the formation of thrombus over the endarterectomy surface.[x] This will be the so-called gray thrombus made up of platelets and fibrin with few red cells. Such a deficit after a normal interval requires immediate exploration for removal of the thrombus covering the endarterectomy surface. Gray thrombus can be easily lifted from the endarterectomy surface which is then irrigated with dextran 40 before closing the arteriostomy with a patch.

Patients who develop a deficit after having aroused from anesthesia with a normal neurologic examination should be returned to the operating room without delay. There is no place here for an emergency duplex scan (US images of a fresh surgical field is poor) or for a CT of the brain without contrast. The latter has sometimes been advised in order to rule out the theoretical possibility of an intracerebral bleed. I have never encountered or heard of such a finding under these circumstances. The delay imposed by the CT may negate the possibility of a full recovery following immediate reexploration and dextran treatment.

In acute stroke the timing for the appearance of lesions in the CT is as follows. Following a large stroke it will take at least 3 hours before any signs of infarction appear. After 24 hours about 60% of the hemispheric infarcts can be seen and, after a week, all the hemispheric infarcts are evident. The first signs of a middle cerebral territory infarct are the obliteration of the lentiform nucleus and the loss of the insular ribbon. Both of these areas are perfused by arteries which are functionally, not anatomically, terminal and cannot be resupplied by collateral flow. The edema that follows ischemic damage obscures the silhouette of the lentiform nucleus and the white-gray ribbon that forms the lateral margin of the insula. As the edema increases, mass effects are evident in the effacement of the sulci and compression of the lateral ventricle.

These early signs of a large hemispheric infarction generally contraindicate an acute intervention for fear that it may result in a more ominous hemorrhagic infarction in the ischemic brain.

A *deficit developing several hours after endarterectomy* requires a brain CT and an arteriogram. The latter may show some unsuspected technical flaw, a thrombosed ICA or, rarely, a thrombosed ECA origin embolizing the ICA.

OPERATIVE RISK DATA

The average risk of carotid endarterectomy in my experience with this procedure (3,538 cases) does not represent the current situation because over time I have modified the indications, techniques, and the anesthesia protocols. The last 1,000 endarterectomies were done under uniform protocols and techniques.

---

[x] I have not seen gray thrombus after CEA since 1990 when we added dextran 40 to the intraoperative carotid protocol.

CAROTID ENDARTERECTOMY (2002 TO 2012)

N	Stroke		Death	
	N	%	*N*	%
1,000	3	0.3	0	0

REFERENCES

1. Berguer R, Sieggreen MY, Lazo A, Hodakowski GT. The silent brain infarct in carotid surgery. *J Vasc Surg.* 1986;3:442–447.
2. Schaller BG. Hypothermia and stroke: the pathophysiological background. *ISP Pathophysiol.* 2003;10: 7–35.
3. Deng H, Han HS, Cheng D, Sun GH, Yenari MA. Mild hypothermia inhibits inflammation after experimental stroke and brain inflammation. *Stroke.* 2003;34:2495–2501.
4. Berguer R. Eversion endarterectomy of the carotid bifurcation. In: Veith F., ed. *Current Critical Problems in Vascular Surgery.* St Louis, MO: Quality Medical Publishing; 1993;441–447.
5. Etheredge. A simple technique for carotid endarterectomy. *Am J Surg.* 1970;1970:275–278.
6. Sessa C, Morasch M, Berguer R, Kline R, Jacobs J, Arden R. Carotid resection and replacement with autogenous arterial graft during operation for neck malignancy. *Ann Vasc Surg.* 1998;12:229–235.
7. Moreau P, Albat B, Thevenet A. Surgical treatment of extracranial internal carotid artery aneurysm. *Ann Vasc Surg.* 1994;8:409–416.
8. Rosset E, Albertini JN, Magnan PE, Ede B, Thomassin JM, Branchereau A. Surgical treatment of extracranial internal carotid artery aneurysms. *J Vasc Surg.* 2000;31:713–723.
9. Zwolak RM, Whitehouse WM Jr, Knake JE, et al. Atherosclerotic extracranial carotid artery aneurysms. *J Vasc Surg.* 1984;1:415–422.
10. Painter AT, Hertzer NR, Beven EG and O'Hara PJ. Extracranial carotid aneurysms: reports of six cases and reviews of the literature. *J Vasc Surg.* 1985;2:312–318.
11. McCann RL. Basic data related to peripheral artery aneurysms. *Ann Vasc Surg.* 1990;4:411–414.
12. Thevenet A. Chirurgie des lesions non atheromateuses carotidiennes. In: Kieffer E, Natali J, eds. *Aspects Techniques de la Chirurgie Carotidienne.* Paris: Editions AERCV, Paris 1987. pp 219–229.

CHAPTER 6

Reconstruction of the Vertebral Artery

INDICATIONS FOR SURGERY

Reconstruction of the VA is indicated in patients with VBI symptoms and appropriate VA lesions. Other than in reconstructions done for extracranial VA aneurysms, I have operated only on two patients with asymptomatic VA lesions: at the beginning of my experience I did a proximal VA transposition in a young woman with severe post-radiation (95%) bilateral VA stenosis and absent posterior communicantes. The other patient had bilateral ICA and VA occlusions and I did a revascularization of a distal VA in preparation for cardiopulmonary bypass. All other VA reconstructions have been done in symptomatic patients in whom the VA lesion was shown, or could be presumed, to be the cause of the neurologic symptoms.

Patients present with either low-flow or embolic symptoms.[i] *Low-flow symptoms* are iterative, caused by the same neck movement (e.g., rotation to one side or extension) and can be reproduced on clinical examination. They do not result in brain infarction. The potential morbidity for these patients is not a stroke but rather the trauma that may follow a bout of vertigo or syncope at an inopportune time (driving, climbing a ladder).

Embolic symptoms, on the contrary, have varied topography depending on where the microembolus impacts and are not triggered by any specific motion. The MRI will show a cerebellar or brain stem infarction. They also have a particularly ominous prognosis: posterior brain infarction is three times more deadly than anterior infarction.

In patients presenting with *low-flow* symptoms secondary to severe VA stenosis, the dominant VA is the one that must be reconstructed. In determining what constitutes a critical reduction of diameter, I have followed the heuristic that 75% of the total inflow needs to be compromised to justify ascribing the symptoms to low flow. This means that a patient with an equivalent VA should have bilateral >75% stenosis in both arteries or, if there is clearly a dominant or single VA, the latter should have >75% of its diameter compromised.

Patients with low-flow symptoms, in addition to their significant VA lesions, have minute or absent posterior communicating arteries. This lack of a compensatory mechanism from the carotid territory potentiates the inflow deficit imposed by the stenotic vertebral lesion. Patients with low-flow VBI secondary to rotation–extension of the neck need to have the cause–effect relationship proven by dynamic

---

[i] In VA dissection the symptoms may be caused by either mechanism.

arteriography (see Section "Dynamic Compression of the Vertebral Artery (Bow Hunter Syndrome)" in Chapter 3).

In patients with *embolic VBI*, the VA responsible for the embolization must be identified (see Section "Divergence vs. Convergence" in Chapter 2) in order to plan treatment. In some cases with bilateral VA disease, the responsible VA can be deduced from the location of the cerebellar infarction. However, when the infarction is in the inferior cerebellar, basilar, or posterior cerebral artery territory and both VAs are patent and diseased, one may not be able to presume what side is causing the symptoms.

The presentation of my experience with VA reconstruction to an audience of clinicians invariably raises the demand for a prospective randomized trial to demonstrate the validity of VA reconstruction. But the known contrasting outcomes of low-flow (physical limitations, trauma) and embolic disease (severe incapacitating stroke or death) render useless any conclusion that could be reached by such a study.

Assume that patients with symptoms of VBI and evidence of severe VA disease are randomized into operative and non-operative therapy. Assume further that we choose the traditional end-points of death and stroke and that the distribution of etiology would be similar to what we see in practice: approximately 70% having low-flow symptoms and 30% embolic symptoms.

As clinical practice dictates today, those patients with VBI induced by rotation of the head (transient low-flow) would not be entered into the study because dynamic arteriography is not part of the clinical workup today and this is the only test that demonstrates the cause–effect relationship between rotation of the head and vertebral flow arrest. Even if their workup were to involve a routine CTA, the latter would fail to show any vertebral lesion. The rest of the patients with low flow would not show any improvement in end-points with surgery because the death/stroke rate in these patients is similar to that of a normal population (their morbidity is limited to some physical disability and to trauma from loss of equilibrium at a critical moment).

Those patients with VBI secondary to embolization that were randomized to surgery would be exposed to a death/stroke risk of <2% once, but the beneficial effects of the operation in this subset will be diluted by the non-effect on death and stroke end-points noted in the larger low-flow group. And in this subset with an embolic etiology, those randomized to medical therapy will experience strokes that have a lethal outcome that is three times greater than is seen in strokes due to carotid disease.

The outcome of such an indiscriminate randomization (not differentiating low-flow from embolic etiologies) would not improve our management of VBI and would likely result in greater disability and death (from those patients with an embolic pathology).

PROXIMAL VERTEBRAL RECONSTRUCTION

Nearly all proximal VA reconstructions are done by *transposing its first segment to the neighboring CCA*. This technique requires only limited dissection, one anastomosis, and has excellent primary patency rates (99% at 5 years).[ii]

[ii] This elegant solution was first described by Roon.[1] My first forays into vertebral reconstruction were SA–VA bypass operations. I switched to the transposition technique shortly afterward[2,3] and it has remained my technique of choice for the correction of V1 lesions.

A roll under the patient's shoulder keeps the head slightly extended and turned to the opposite side with its weight well supported by padding. The incision is S-shaped 6 to 7 cm long. The flaps of the wound are undermined three-fourth of an inch and the two bellies of the sternomastoid muscle are separated (Fig. 6.1A). The omohyoid muscle is divided. The IJV is retracted laterally with the vagus nerve. The CCA is exposed extending its dissection proximally into the mediastinum.

On the left side, the thoracic duct is identified as it emerges behind the carotid turning toward the jugulo-subclavian venous confluent. The duct is ligated and cut (Fig. 6.1B). On the right side, it is common to encounter one or two small lymph ducts that are likewise individually ligated and divided. The next landmark to look for is the vertebral vein (Fig. 6.1C) because the VA will generally be found posterior to it. The vertebral vein follows a similar course to the VA that lies posterior to it. The vein, which is slightly larger than the artery, has a straight trajectory, while the corresponding first segment of the VA can be tortuous and loop upon itself. The vein has branches; the V1 segment of the artery does not. At times, the VA is not found after dividing the vertebral vein. This situation arises with three anatomical variants: (1) when the VA exits the SA more lateral, distal to the level of origin of the internal mammary artery, (2) when the VA exits the posterior wall of the SA and runs transversely to enter, abnormally, the cervical spine at the level of C7, and (3) when the Lt VA enters the cervical spine at C5 or C4, as it does when it takes origin directly from the arch.

As the VA is dissected, the intermediate ganglion is found resting on it. The sympathetic chain that links the intermediate and the stellate ganglia crosses obliquely the VA (Fig. 6.1D). The inferior thyroid artery is divided as it crosses the field transversely entering a fenestration of the sympathetic chain. The VA is dissected from its origin to its disappearance under the lower edge of the longus colli muscle at C6. Under this musculotendinous edge, there is a vein that crosses over the VA and should be controlled with bipolar cautery. The midportion of V1 is freed from the overlying intermediate ganglion without severing the rami that exit the ganglion medially and laterally.

After adequate heparinization, the VA is occluded at the level of the longus colli with a Heifitz or a Schwartz microclip. The origin of the VA is suture ligated close to its origin and then divided placing a hemoclip on the stump for added security. Once the artery is divided, it is pulled through the sympathetic ring that surrounds it (Fig. 6.1D) at the level of the intermediate ganglion and is brought next to the CCA to verify that it will reach with ease the site planned for transposition. Damage to the intermediate ganglion or its rami will result in an incomplete Horner's (ptosis and miosis, but no anhydrosis). The approximate site for transposition to the posterior wall of CCA is marked with a pen.

If there is a tongue of the ostial plaque still present in the distal free end of the VA, a very short, superficial, eversion endarterectomy will remove this fragment of the plaque.

To facilitate the anastomosis, the CCA is rotated to bring the posterior wall into a lateral position (Fig. 6.1E). The artery is then occluded with a baby Satinsky clamp that allows the assistant to hold the CCA next to the VA during the anastomosis. The arteriostomy in the CCA wall is made with a 5 mm aortic punch and the VA is anastomosed to it with an oblique end-to-side junction with 7-0 polypropylene. After proper forward and back bleeding flow is restored into the distal carotid and distal VA.

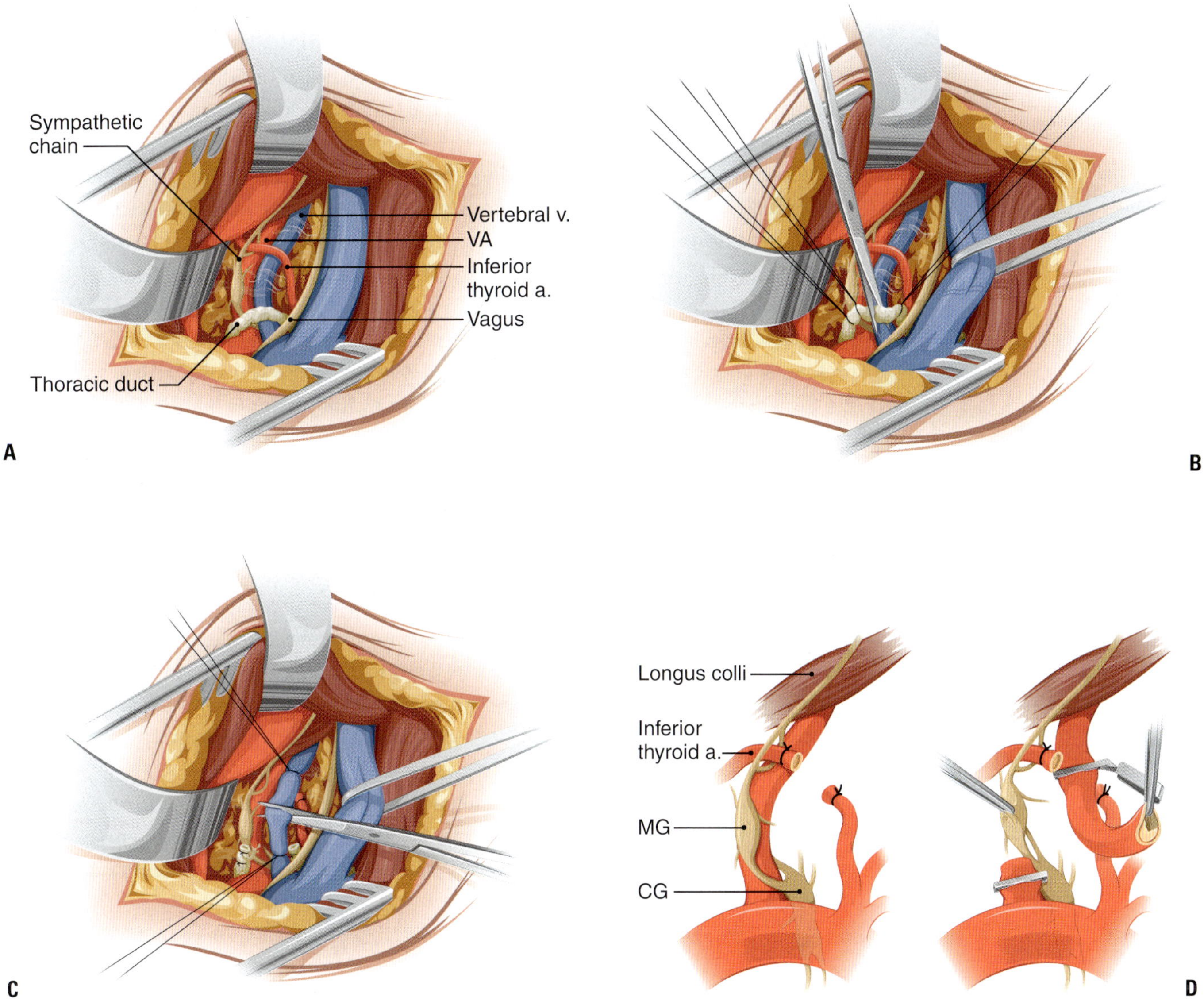

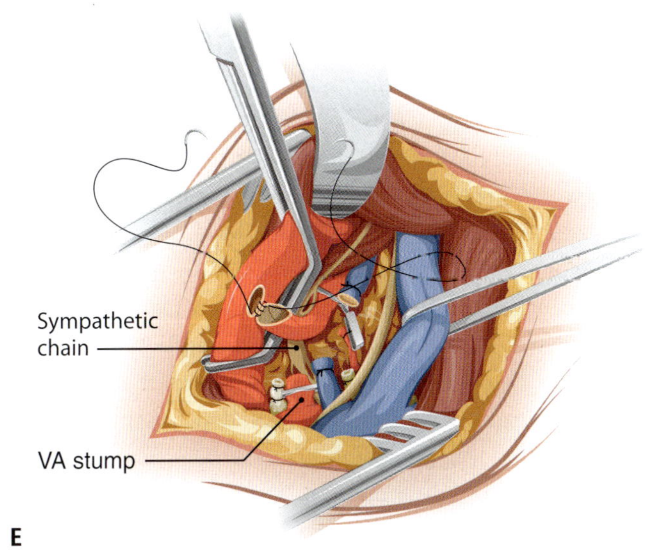

FIGURE 6.1. (**A**) The anatomic elements of the supraclavicular approach to V1. (**B**) Division of the thoracic duct as it emerges from behind the CCA to empty in the jugulo-subclavian confluent. (**C**) Division of the vertebral vein. (**D**) Extricating the VA from the middle ganglion and sympathetic chain. (**E**) Anastomosis of the VA to the posterior wall of the CCA.

When the quality of the neighboring CCA is inadequate to transpose the VA to it, the reconstruction of the latter can be based on the ipsilateral SA by means of a *subclavian vertebral bypass.*[2,3] This alternative may be needed in those cases where the VA enters the transverse process of C7 and the length of available artery is insufficient to reach the CCA.

Reconstruction of the VA based on the SA requires exposure of the second portion of the latter. For this the incision is parallel to the clavicle. The clavicular head of the sternomastoid muscle is cut close to its insertion in the clavicle. The omohyoid muscle is divided and the prescalene fat pad is dissected along its superior, medial, and inferior edges and flipped away from the dissection field leaving lateral attachments as a hinge. The phrenic nerve, which runs on the surface of the scalenus anticus muscle, is gently dissected from the latter. Division of the scalenus anticus exposes the SA which is dissected for the length needed to find the best site for clamping it. Medially, the VA is isolated in a fashion similar to the one described above for its transposition. The distal anastomosis is done first.

The proximal VA is divided and suture ligated. If there is enough artery above the intermediate ganglion, the artery may be divided immediately above the ganglion to avoid dissecting around it. The distal end of the VA should be no less than 1.5 cm from the lower edge of the longus colli muscle to have secure control of the VA below this muscle. The artery is spatulated to construct the anastomosis to the saphenous vein graft. Once the distal anastomosis is completed, attention is turned to the SA. A baby Satinsky clamp is best suited to control the SA. The arteriostomy in the superior wall of the SA is made with a 5 mm aortic punch, and the graft is trimmed to appropriate length and is anastomosed to the SA.

If an adequate vein graft is not available and there is a redundancy in the proximal VA, the artery may be cut close to its origin in the SA and brought to a more lateral site to be transposed to it. This site could be the stump of an amputated thyrocervical trunk.

DISTAL VERTEBRAL RECONSTRUCTION

The reconstruction of the distal VA can be accomplished through different techniques: the most frequent choice is a vein bypass from the CCA (Fig. 6.2). Other options (Fig. 6.3) are transposition of the ECA to the VA, transposition of the occipital artery to the VA, and transposition of the VA to the high cervical ICA.[4]

For all these options the *exposure of V3 at the C1–C2 level is the common pathway.* The choice for this site is based on several advantages. There is more length of VA accessible between these two transverse processes than at any other intervertebral level, facilitating control and anastomosis of the artery at this level. The level of C1–C2 is also distal to most sites where the VA may be compressed by osteophytes so, in a neck involved with generalized osteoarthrosis, the bypass corrects the primary compression site demonstrated in V2, as well as jump over additional, more distal, compression sites that may exist. Most relevant, C1–C2 is the level at which the VA reconstitutes when its intracervical (V2) course has occluded. At this level, branches from the occipital artery or cervical ascending artery enter the VA and preserve patency of its V3 and V4 segments, thus making it available for surgical revascularization.[5,6]

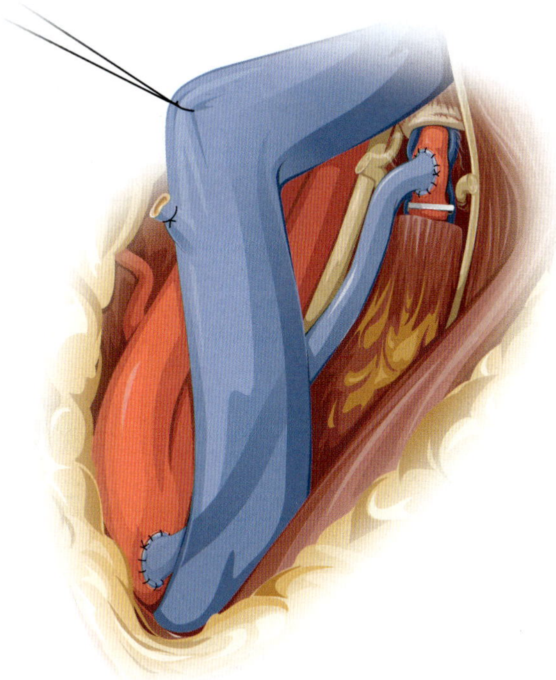

FIGURE 6.2. A standard CCA–distal VA bypass.

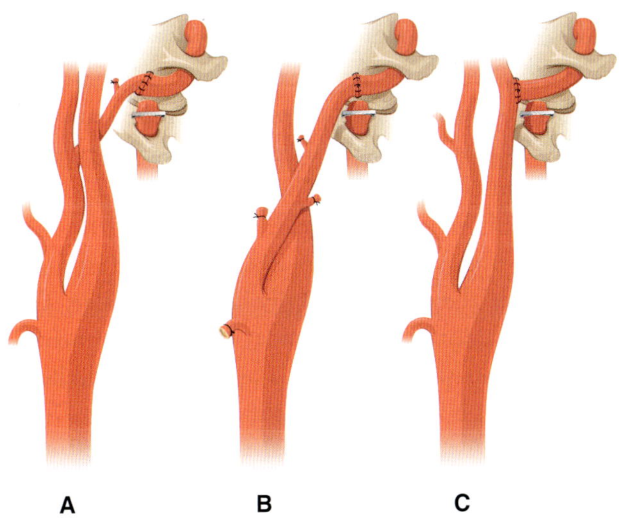

FIGURE 6.3. Other options for revascularization of the distal VA at V3: (**A**) occipital to V3 transposition, (**B**) ECA–V3 transposition, and (**C**) V3–ICA transposition.

The patient has his head turned toward the opposite side. The earlobe has been stitched anteriorly in case the incision has to be carried up to the mastoid. The incision is similar to the one used for carotid endarterectomy (Fig. 6.4). The external jugular vein is divided. The tip of the carotid gland is elevated. The greater auricular nerve may be mobilized and moved aside, or it may need to be divided. Dissection proceeds

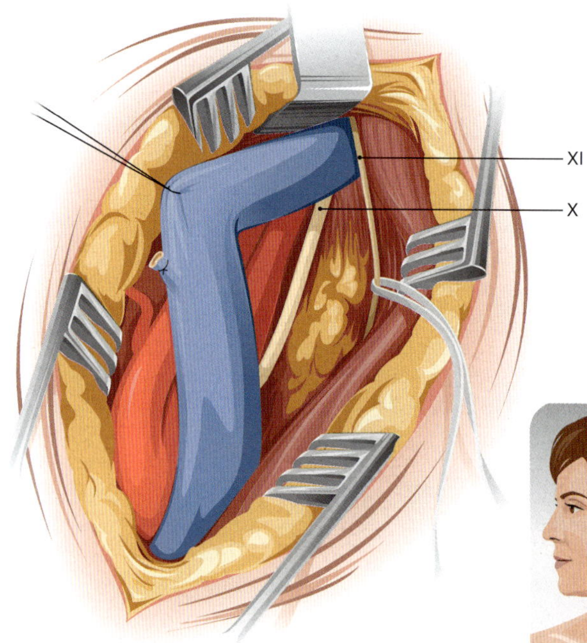

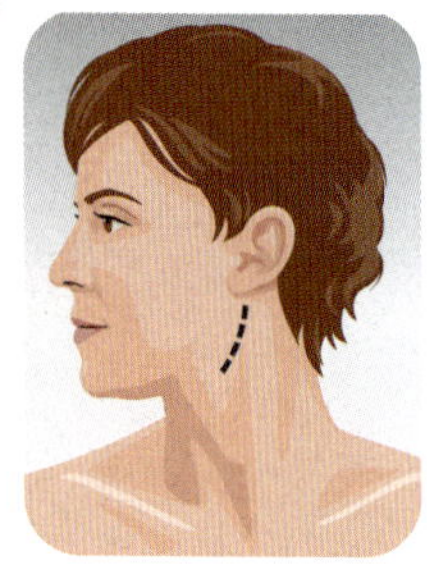

FIGURE 6.4. Incision and approach to the distal VA.

posterior to the jugular vein between it and the sternomastoid muscle (Fig. 6.5A–G). The accessory spinal nerve emerges below the edge of the sternomastoid muscle at 2½ fingerbreadths below the mastoid process. The nerve is freed from the retrojugular fatty tissue and dissected under the digastric muscle until the surgeon can feel the nerve crossing over the sharp boney prominence of the transverse process of C1. At this point, the IJV is found interposed between the XI nerve and the transverse process. The digastric muscle is divided. The transverse process of C1 once exposed will be the upper limit of the operative field. The blade of the automatic retractor, if one is used, is placed immediately above it. Clearing the fatty tissue that overlies the levator scapula muscle allows us to identify its anterior edge. The anterior ramus of C2 exits under this anterior edge and divides into three branches. The upper and lower ones are loops that anastomose with C1 and C3, the middle one is the proper C2 ramus. Once the ramus is identified, a right angle clamp is slid over it lifting the levator muscle which is then cut with cautery 1 to 2 cm from its insertion at C1. The distal stump of muscle and tendon attached to C1 is removed with scissors to expose the boney prominence of the transverse process.

The C2 ramus bulges out as it crosses over the VA that runs perpendicular to it. The ramus is cut on top of the VA and its two ends are held separately by weighted sutures. The VA can be seen with the vertebral veins running along its anterior and posterior walls. The dissection of the artery is delicate and necessitates fine bipolar coagulation to control the vertebral veins. The VA is exposed from the top of C2 to the bottom of C1. Occasionally, if one runs short of exposed length, it may be necessary to resect the anterior edge of the transverse process of C1 by clearing the process of any muscle or tendon. The VA is looped avoiding injury to any collateral that may be entering it postero-medially. After heparinization the artery is prepared for anastomosis by using a specially designed baby J-clamp that has a gentle bite and the

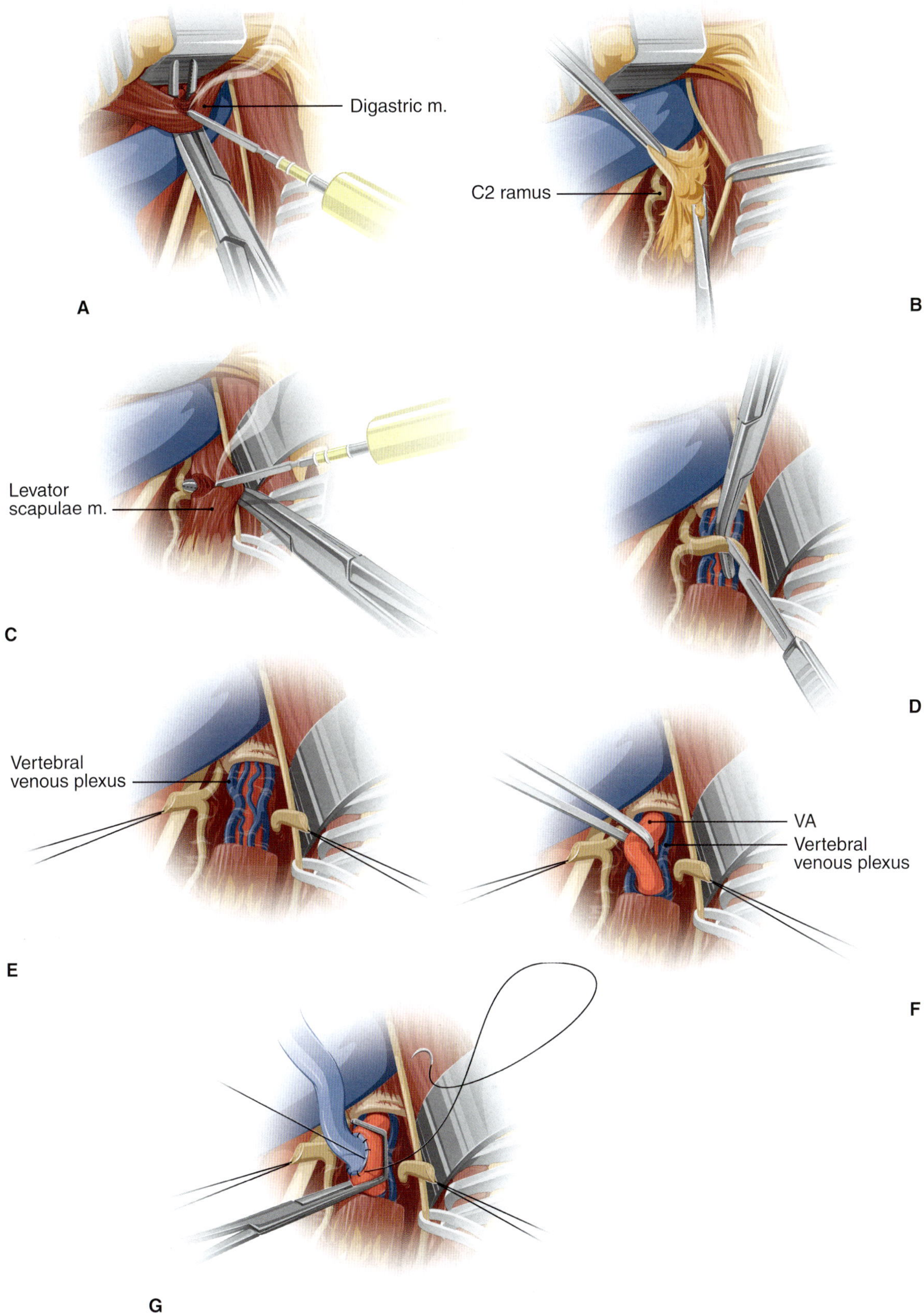

FIGURE 6.5. Isolation of the distal VA at the C1–C2 interspace: (**A**) division of the digastrics muscle, (**B**) removal of fibrofatty tissue covering the levator muscle, (**C**) division of the levator muscle, (**D**) cutting the ramus of C2 to (**E**) exposure of the underlying VA with its accompanying venous plexus, and (**F**) isolation of the VA for the distal anastomosis (**G**) of the bypass graft.

appropriate length to stay away from the surgeon while securing the artery in place. The VA here has a thinner wall than in its first segment.[iii]

Common Carotid to Distal (V3) Vertebral Bypass

The harvested vein is marked with a blue pen to avoid axial twisting. The distal anastomosis is done first (Fig. 6.5G). An angulated baby J-clamp occludes the VA and an end-to-side anastomosis is performed in an open fashion with 7-0 polypropylene and a small needle (BV175). A tunnel under the IJV brings the proximal end of the graft next to the selected side for implantation in the CCA. The graft is anastomosed to the CCA on its lateral wall (Fig. 6.2).

Absent a good segment of saphenous vein, a bypass can be constructed by everting a segment of occluded ICA and using it as a free autograft (Fig. 6.6). There may be calcification or disease in the CCA that would disqualify this site for proximal insertion of the graft. The available and suitable saphenous vein segment may also be too short to reach proximally the CCA. In either of these two cases, the ECA may provide a good source of inflow (Figs. 6.7 and 6.8) avoiding the need to interrupt flow in the ICA.

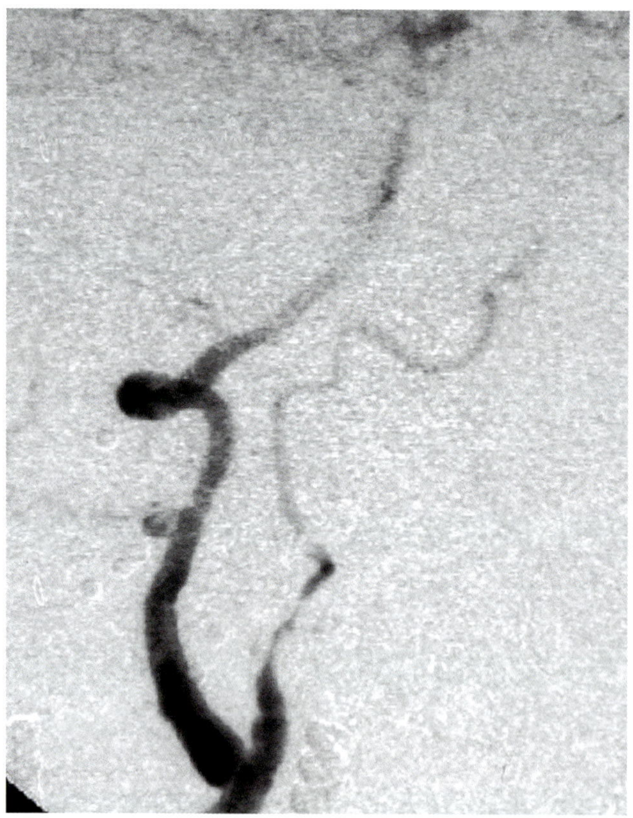

FIGURE 6.6. Distal VA bypass constructed with a segment of occluded ICA that was cleared by eversion endarterectomy for its use as a free graft.

[iii] Its wall thickness is about one-third of that of the saphenous vein graft that will be anastomosed to it.

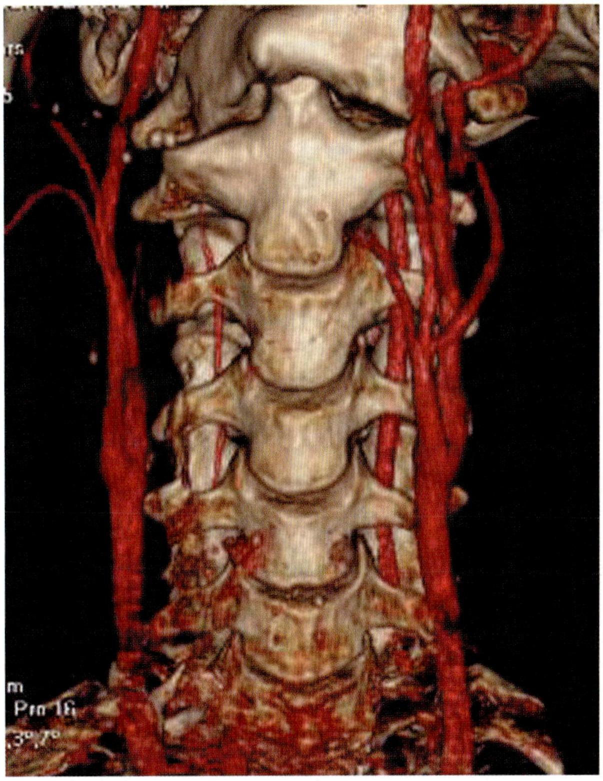

FIGURE 6.7A. A Lt distal VA vein bypass taking origin in the Lt ECA.

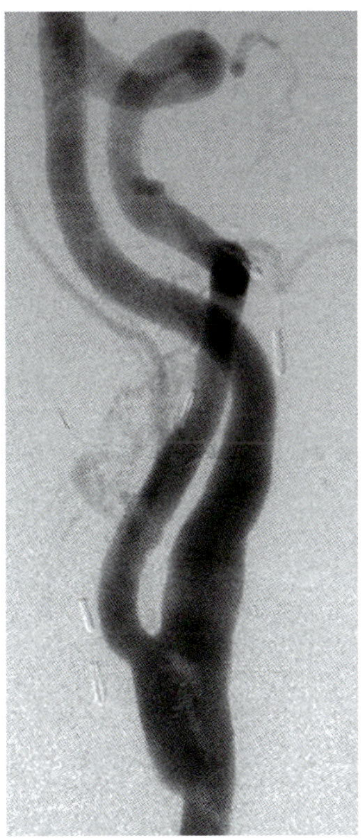

FIGURE 6.7B. A vein bypass from the ECA ostium to the distal VA.

Transposition of External Carotid to Distal (V3) Vertebral Artery

The suitability of the ECA to be the supply for the distal VA is established preoperatively in the CTA or arteriogram. This includes showing that its origin is free of plaque and that its pattern of branching will provide a trunk of appropriate diameter to be anastomosed to the distal VA. If the ECA has a pattern of early branching, it may not be possible to end up with a single trunk of sufficient diameter for its transposition to the VA.

The ECA is skeletonized up to its division into superficial temporal and maxillary branches. The superior thyroid artery is divided to permit the counterclock rotation of the bifurcation that will result in the origin of the ECA being posterior to the bifurcation (Fig. 6.8). The distal end of the ECA is divided and its distal stump is suture ligated. The proximal opening of the ECA is cleared of adventitia in preparation for its end-to-side anastomosis to the distal VA. A metal clip placed in the VA immediately below the anastomosis transforms the end-to-side into a functional end-to-end junction (Fig. 6.9).

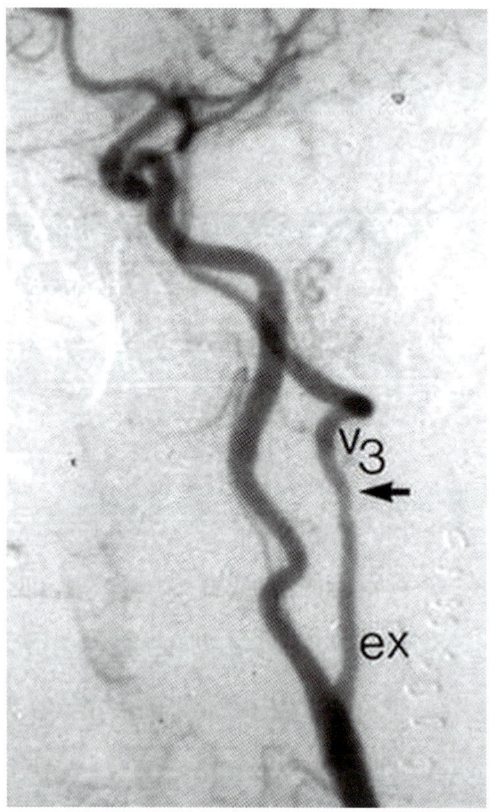

FIGURE 6.8. Postop agram after transposition of the ECA to the distal VA. The 180 degree rotation of the carotid bifurcation leaves the ICA as the anterior component of the bifurcation. By this maneuver, the ECA can more easily reach V3. Arrow points to distal anastomosis, below C1 transverse foramen.

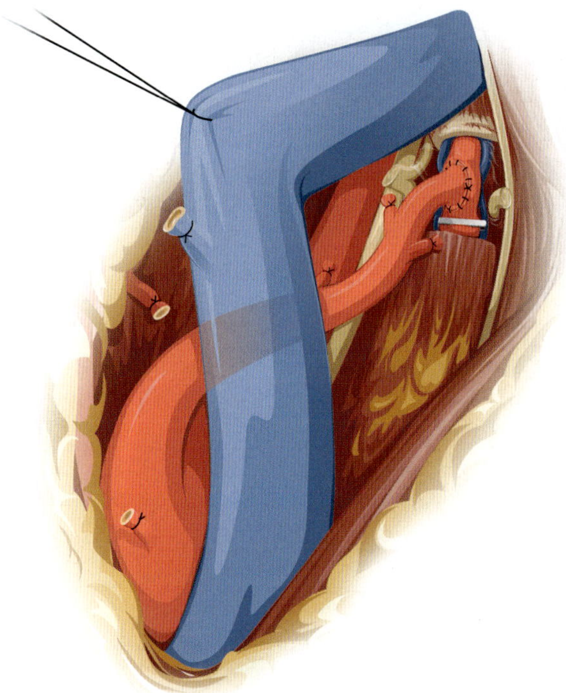

FIGURE 6.9. Transposition of the ECA to the distal VA.

Transposition of Occipital to Distal (V3) Vertebral Artery

It is unusual to encounter an occipital artery that, as a collateral, has grown to a diameter adequate to match that of the VA. I have only encountered such enlarged occipital arteries in patients who have had an occipital collateral supplying a VA for a long time, such as in children whose proximal VA was included in the subclavian flap used to correct an aortic coarctation. When the occipital artery is so enlarged, the revascularization of the distal VA can be accomplished by transposing the occipital artery to it (Fig. 6.3A). The surgical exposure for this operation is limited to the territory above the hypoglossal nerve. The occipital artery will be found running underneath and parallel to the digastric muscle. Two small branches that the occipital artery sends to the digastric muscle are ligated. The occipital artery is dissected far enough to reach the exposed distal VA below it. The anastomosis between the two is constructed with 7-0 polypropylene.

Transposition of Distal (V3) Vertebral Artery to Upper Cervical Internal Carotid Artery

This technique should not be used in patients who have an occluded contralateral ICA because of the need to clamp the ipsilateral ICA during the reconstruction. For this procedure, the distal VA is exposed at the C1–C2 interval in the standard manner described above. The upper cervical ICA is found anterior to the VA at this level

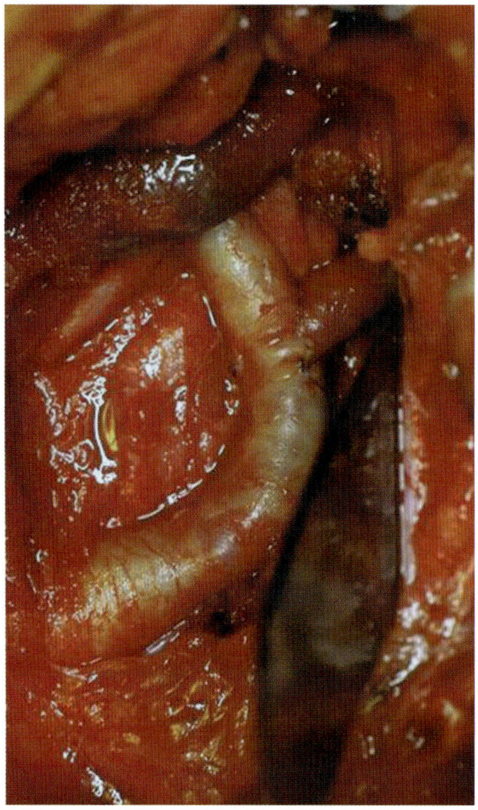

FIGURE 6.10. The distal VA has been transposed to the posterior wall of the ICA.

and is freed for a length of 2 cm. The VA is freed down to the transverse process of C2 where its proximal end will be divided and suture ligated. The distal VA is then brought anteriorly into proximity with the ICA. The arteriotomy in the ICA is made in its posterior wall and the distal VA is anastomosed to it end-to-side with 7-0 polypropylene (Fig. 6.10).

In some instances where the VA is too short to reach the ICA easily, an "H" type of bypass can be done by inserting a short autogenous graft (ECA or saphenous vein) first into the VA and last into the ICA.

SUBOCCIPITAL APPROACH TO THE VERTEBRAL ARTERY AT C0–C1

The VA needs to be exposed in its suboccipital segment in patients who occlude the VA when they rotate or extend their neck, by compressing it between the occipital bone and the lamina of the atlas. Exposure at this level is also useful in the rare instance of a symptomatic VA dissection that extends to the level of C1 and does not respond to heparin.[7] In this approach, the artery is isolated in its pars atlantica,[iv] as it rests on the posterior lamina of C1, before it enters the foramen magnum (Fig. 6.11).

[iv] The idea for this approach came from a drawing in Kirtschner's classic *Textbook of Operative Surgery* (Fig. 6.12) published in 1930.

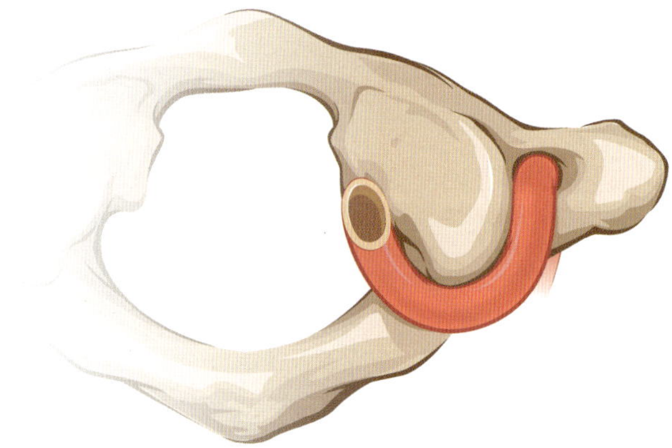

FIGURE 6.11. The *pars atlantica* of the VA.

The patient is in the park bench or prone position.[7] The incision is suboccipital, horizontal from the midline to the mastoid tip where it turns down following the posterior edge of the SM muscle (Fig. 6.13A–F). Trapezius, semispinalis, and splenius capiti muscle are cut. The SM muscle is deinserted and reflected down. The IJV and the XI nerve are identified and protected. The transverse process and the sharp edge of the lamina of C1

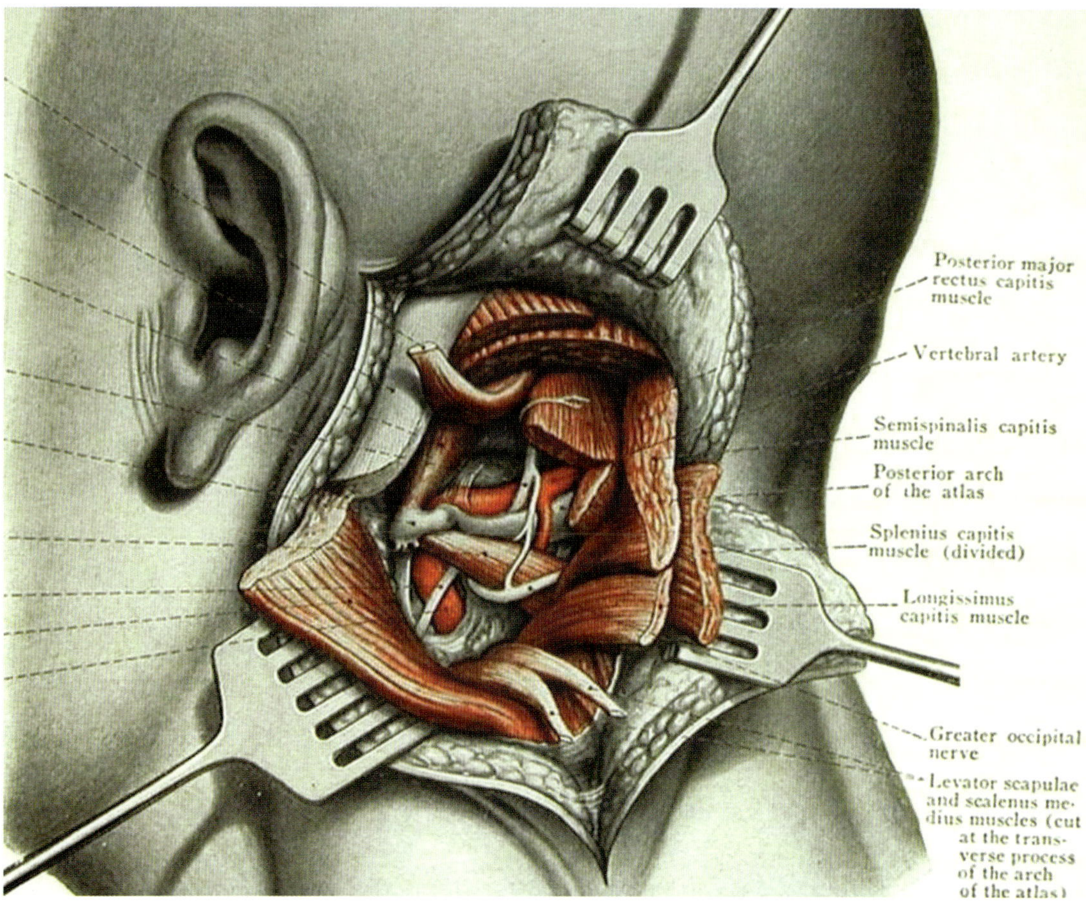

FIGURE 6.12. Illustration in Kirshner's textbook.

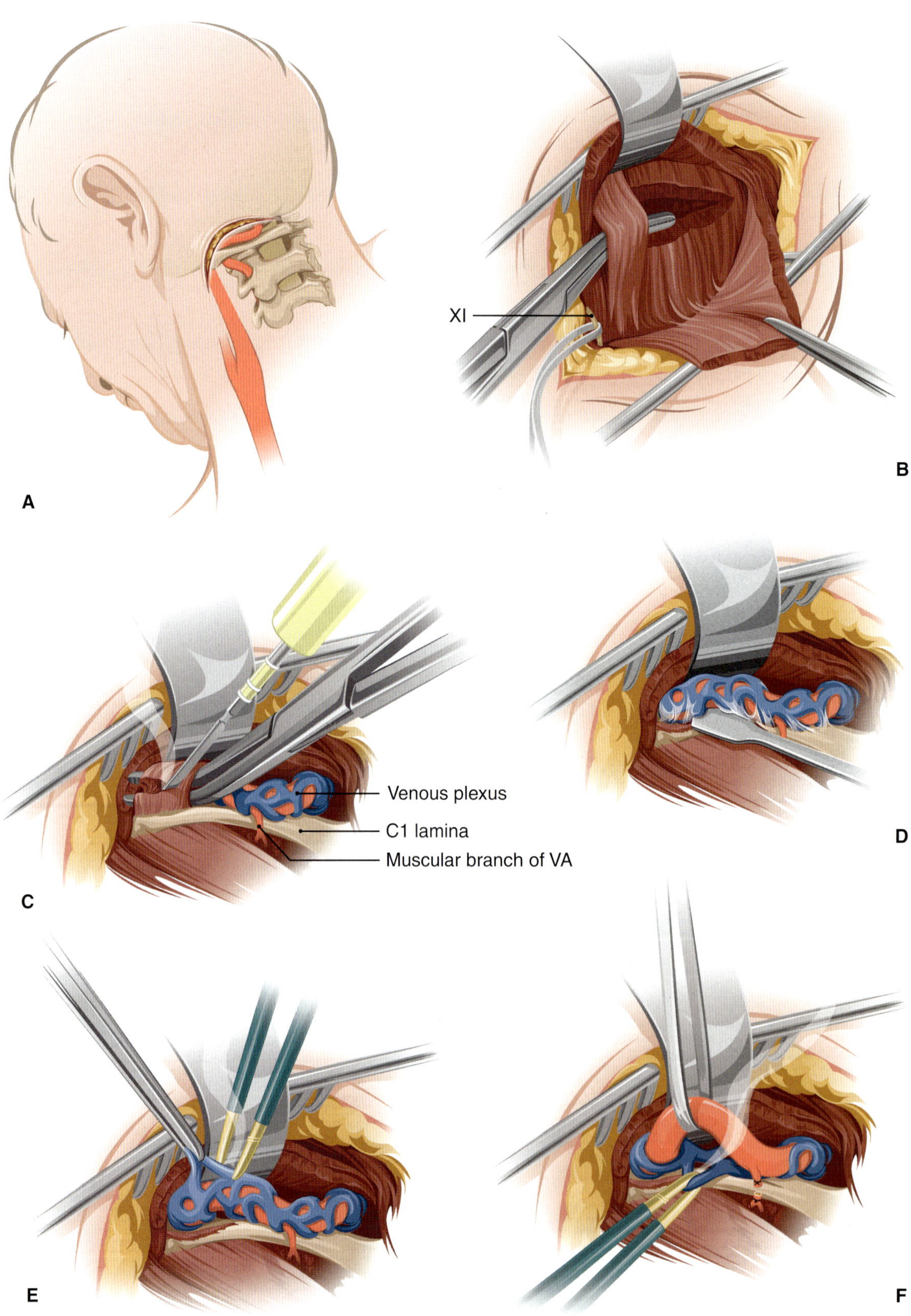

FIGURE 6.13. Steps for the suboccipital approach to the VA: (**A**) incision, (**B**) division of nuchal muscles, (**C**) exposure of the VA covered by a venous plexus, (**D**) lifting the VA from the lamina, (**E**) bipolar coagulation control of the plexus, and (**F**) the pars atlantica isolated.

can be felt by palpation. The short suboccipital muscles (obliquus capitis, rectus capitis) are divided and the artery is exposed below them covered by a plexus of veins. The artery is anchored inferiorly by a muscular branch that keeps the VA tented down and perching over the lamina. Once this branch is divided, the VA can be lifted away from the lamina. Control of the veins surrounding the VA is achieved with bipolar electrocoagulation.

When approached posteriorly in this manner, the distal cervical ICA runs medial to the SM muscle in a trough whose sides are the mastoid and jaw laterally and the cervical spine medially. The ICA is flanked laterally by the IJV and covered by the cranial nerves IX, X, and XI. The carotid is isolated in the last 3 cm of its course before it enters the temporal canal. The vein graft is tended between the ICA and the VA over the posterior lamina of C1 that does not need to be resected if the bypass is performed to revascularize a VA that is occluded or dissected below C1 (Fig. 6.14).

When the indication for surgery is that a patient experiences VBI symptoms when the angiogram shows the compression of the VA between the occipital bone and the atlas, the aim of the operation is simply to resect the lamina that functions here as the lower element of bone compression on the artery (Fig. 6.15A and B). For this, the lamina needs to be freed of muscular attachments and the VA must be lifted away from it. The surfaces of the lamina are freed with a Key periosteal elevator. The VA is lifted and protected behind a small soft malleable retractor. When the ventral aspect of the lamina is being freed, there will be bleeding from the epidural venus plexus that can be controlled by elevating the head of the bed, continuous irrigation/suction, and the use of cotonoids. With the VA protected by the retractor, the lamina is first divided with a high speed drill and the two ends are resected with rongeur and Kerrison cutters till 2 cm of lamina have been removed (Fig. 6.15). In a case of recurrent

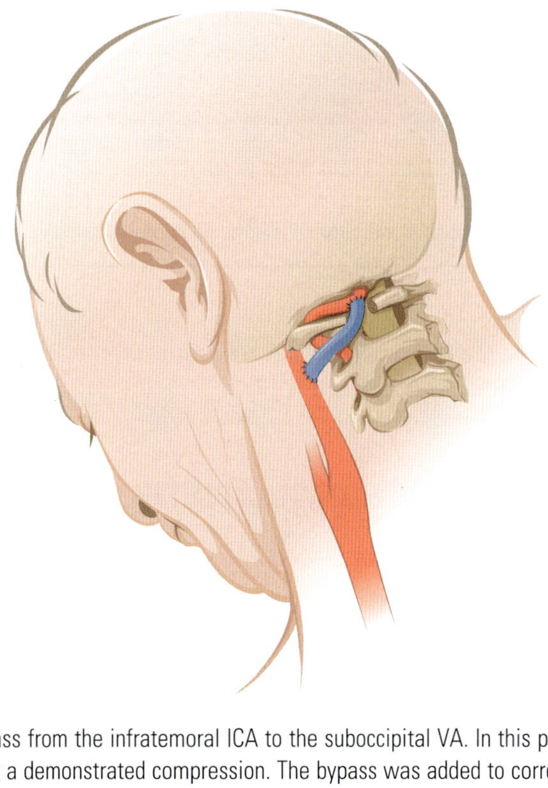

FIGURE 6.14. Bypass from the infratemoral ICA to the suboccipital VA. In this patient the laminectomy was done to correct a demonstrated compression. The bypass was added to correct a severely diseased VA at the site of compression.

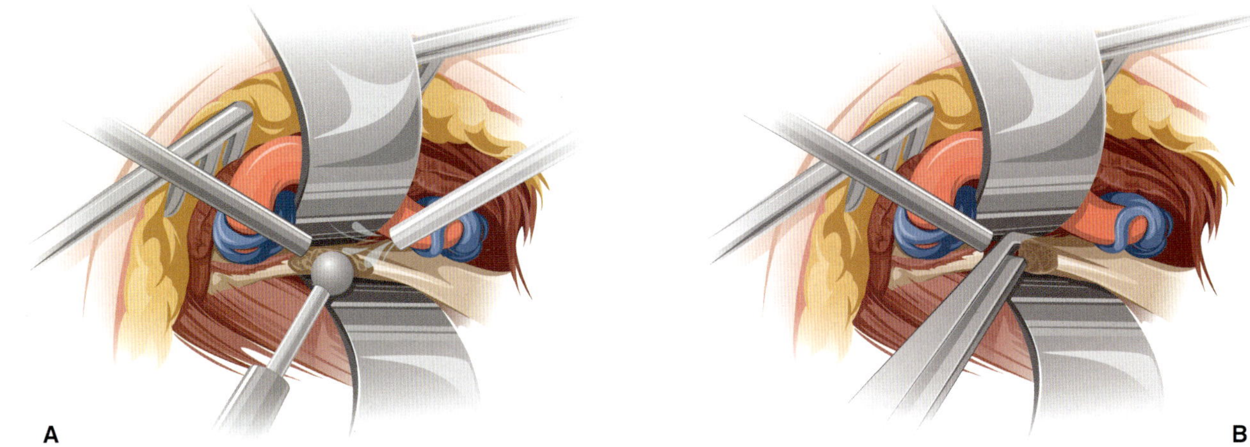

FIGURE 6.15. Partial laminectomy of C1.

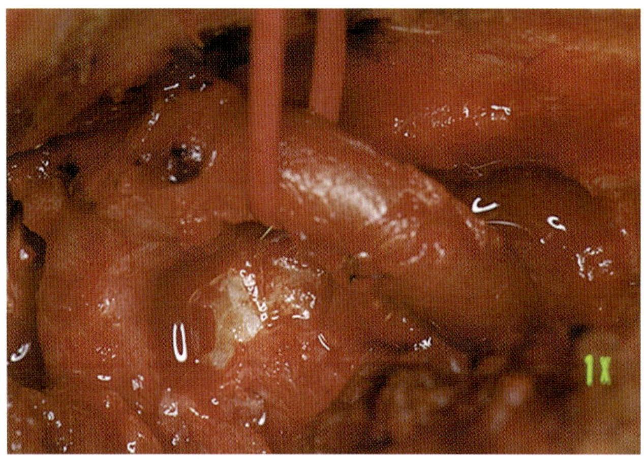

FIGURE 6.16. The *pars atlantica* is lifted. In this patient with recurrent compression at C0-C1 the transverse process of C1 has also been removed from the vertical portion of the VA on the left side of the picture. To the right, the VA disappears under the rongeured edge of the foramen magnum.

compression, most likely due to an inadequate laminectomy, additional bone (C1) may need to be removed (Figs. 6.16 and 6.17).

RESECTION OF VERTEBRAL ANEURYSMS

Access and control of an *extracranial VA aneurysm* is difficult. The fact that both VAs converge into the BA precludes the use of Hunterian ligation (Fig. 6.18). To thrombose a VA aneurysm, the latter must be trapped between a proximal and distal ligature. If the patient has an aplastic contralateral VA, ligation of the VA bearing the aneurysm is a risky procedure. In fact it is risky even when the opposite VA is patent and normally connected to the BA: there are case reports in the neurosurgical literature[8] where ligation of a VA resulted in progression of the thrombus into the BA with subsequent brain infarction and death.

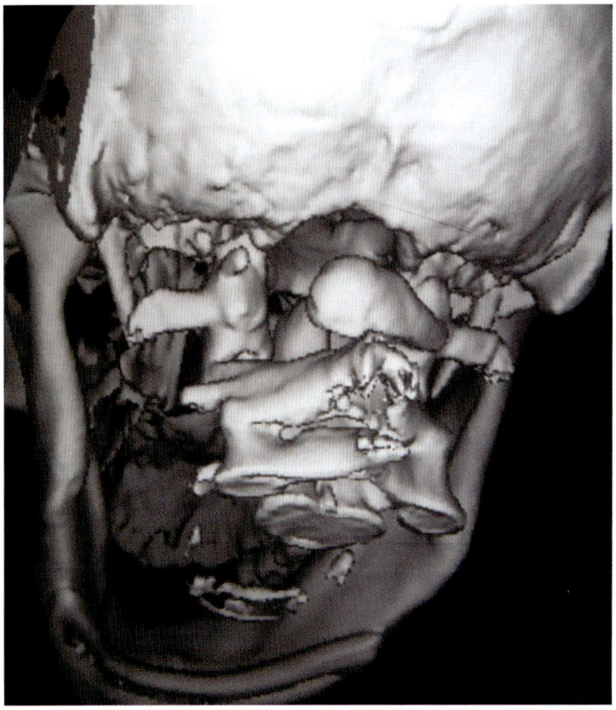

FIGURE 6.17. Postop CT on the same patient (Fig. 6.16) showing the Lt hemilaminectomy and resected transverse process of C1.

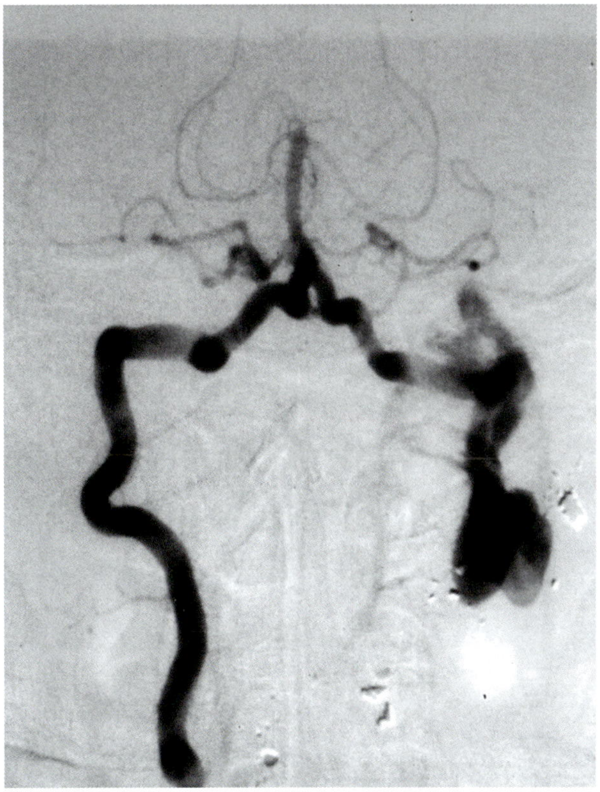

FIGURE 6.18. Proximal ligation of Lt VA aneurysm failed to avoid continued pressurization of it from the opposite VA.

Eight of the nine primary VA aneurysms that we have seen were treated surgically. The reconstruction was a CCA–V3 bypass in six, aneurysmorraphy and vertebral AVF repair in one, and proximal and distal ligation in one. In this last patient with Ehler-Danlos, three attempts to do the distal anastomosis (to V3) failed by tears along the suture line and the distal VA was ligated. This difficulty in suturing vessels in patients with Ehler-Danlos disease justifies our preference for endovascular trapping avoiding a reconstruction.

REOPERATIONS

In most reoperations in the distal VA, the restenosis has occurred in the distal anastomosis. A critical point of the reoperation is dissecting, resecting, and redoing the distal anastomosis. The best surgical sequence has been to isolate the failing bypass in its mid-portion and to continue the dissection around its adventitia until it disappears under the transverse process of C1. The transverse process is then devoided of periosteum and scar and its anterior portion is resected using a combination of rongeur and Kerrison cutter. The isolation of the artery in its course through the transverse process is facilitated by the fact that most of the periarterial venous plexus has been coagulated in the previous operation. If, for lack of adequate length of available artery intravascular occlusion of the distal VA needs to be carried out, a #2 balloon inserted no further than 1 cm beyond C1 can be used. Inflating a balloon beyond the atlanto-occipital membrane at the level of the foramen magnum may perforate or rupture the thin wall of the V4 segment of the VA (see next section).

REVIEW OF TECHNICAL FAILURES

Early in my distal VA experience I had a patient thrombose a distal vertebral bypass due to a faulty distal anastomosis. At reoperation 24 hours later I took down the anastomosis and noticed the distal VA was occluded with fresh thrombus. I inserted a #2 embolectomy catheter and advanced it for 3 cm to retrieve the thrombus followed by good back flow. The new vein graft was anastomosed and, upon resumption of flow, the patient developed intractable hypertension. When anesthesia was discontinued, the patient was found to be comatose. Post-mortem revealed a *perforation of the V4 segment of the VA caused by the embolectomy catheter* resulting in fatal subarachnoid hemorrhage.

The use of *shunts* in the VA is to be proscribed. The trauma caused by the shunt is likely to destroy the VA and, what's more relevant, a shunt is not needed if adequate measures of cerebral protection are undertaken.

Lymphatic ducts must be ligated to avoid the development of a lymphocele. Avoid suture ligature of the thoracic duct, or any accessory thoracic duct that may be found on the right side, in favor of their double ligature/clipping. Inappropriate ligation of the proximal segment of the thoracic duct as it emerges from the mediastinum posterior to the CCA may result in a chylothorax. This complication will require a thoracotomy for a more proximal ligation of the thoracic duct.

Damage to the rami entering the anterior and posterior edges of the middle cervical ganglion will result in an *incomplete Horner's* syndrome.

An ECA to distal VA transposition follows a more horizontal course than the conventional common carotid to distal VA bypass and its geometry may change with rotation of the neck. Because of this, it is important to avoid *errors in the length of the ECA* that may cause either tenting and tension of the anastomosis when short, or redundancy and kink when too long. All things being equal a carotid to distal VA bypass is preferable to a transposition of the ECA.

The anastomosis to the distal VA is best done as an end-to-side anastomosis. In the early experience with distal VA bypasses I was dividing the VA above C2 and anastomosing its distal free end to the graft. This technique was more likely to result in disturbance of the distal anastomosis by axial rotation of either of its two components.

The development of intimal hyperplasia of the distal anastomosis may be managed by balloon angioplasty (Fig. 6.19) although recurrence at the same site is frequent. In rare occasions when doing the arteriotomy in the distal VA one may find a flap from a more proximal dissection. The extreme thinness of the flap precludes any reattachment to the wall. In the 2 cases where I encountered a dissection flap I have fenestrated the dissection by excising whatever length of flap can be reached within the clamped distal VA.

A specific kind of *reflex sympathetic dystrophy (RSD) of the face* may be observed in patients who had *extensive surgical dissection of the ECA*, such as during a transposition of the ECA to the distal VA or when *lifting the parotid gland* during dissection of the ECA and ICA above the hypoglossal nerve.[9] These patients may develop exquisitely sharp facial pain involving the cheek and hemimandible, triggered by the beginning of mastication or by swallowing citric drinks. This hyperpathic pain can

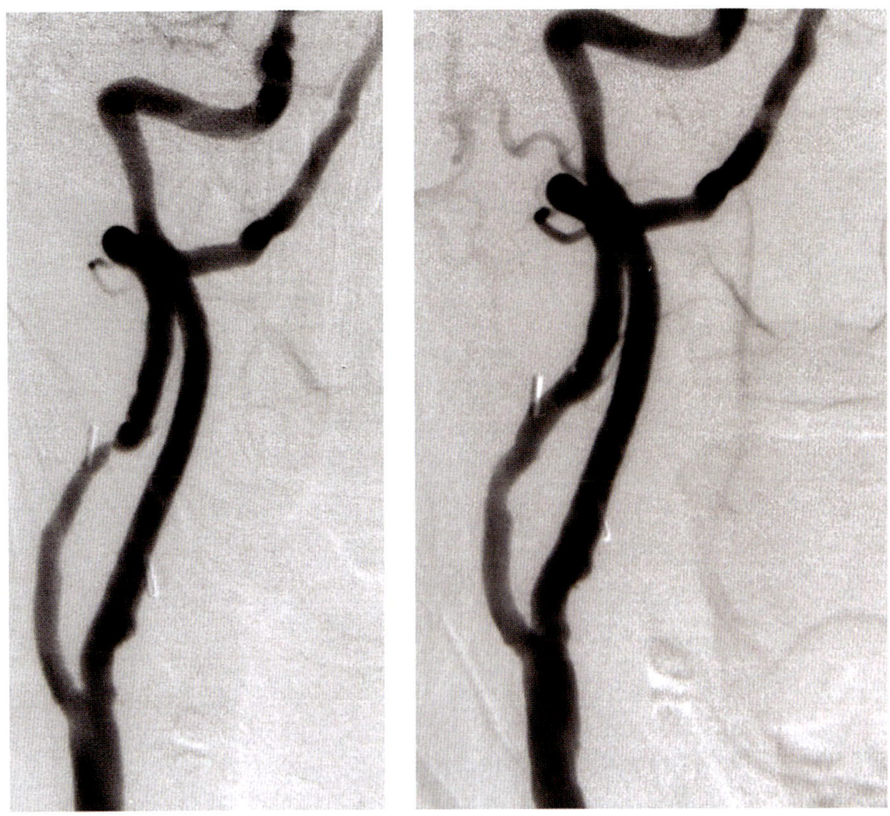

FIGURE 6.19. (**A**) Intimal hyperplasia at the distal anastomosis of an ECA–distal VA transposition appearing 1 year postop. (**B**) Correction by angioplasty.

also be triggered by light stimuli such as shaving. It is not associated with increased sweating or vasomotor changes in the face, as we see in RSD of the extremities. The pain is caused by injury to the post-ganglionic sympathetic fibers that accompany the ECA (to transpose the ECA to the distal VA, the entire length of the former is dissected and skeletonized). The distribution of pain follows, unlike that originating from preganglionic fibers, the dermatome distribution of the corresponding radicular nerve. This RSD of the face has a good prognosis with conservative management consisting of non-neurolytic stellate ganglion blocks that are effective, even when started as a delayed treatment.

OPERATIVE RISK DATA (1980 TO 2011)

	N	Death		Stroke		Death·stroke	
		N	%	*N*	%	*N*	%
Proximal[a]	417	0	0	0	0	0	0
Distal	243	4	1.6	5	2.1	4	2.1
Total	660	4	0.6	5	0.8	5	0.8

[a] Proximal VA reconstructions not done in combination with carotid endarterectomy.

REFERENCES

1. Roon AJ, Ehrenfeld WB, Cooke PB, Wylie EJ. Vertebral Artery Reconstruction. *Am J Surg.* 1979;138:29–36.
2. Berguer R, Bauer R. Vertebral artery bypass. *Arch Surg.* 1976;111:976–979.
3. Berguer R. Vertebral artery reconstruction. *Ann Surg.* 1981;193:441–447.
4. Berguer R, Morasch MD, Kline RA. A review of 100 consecutive reconstructions of the distal vertebral artery for embolic and hemodynamic disease. *J Vasc Surg.* 1998;27:852–859.
5. Berguer R. Distal vertebral artery bypass: techniques, the "occipital connection" and potential use. *J Vasc Surg.* 1985;2:621–626.
6. Berguer R, Kline R, Caplan L. Surgical reconstriuction of the extracranial vertebral artery: management and outcome. *J Vasc Surg.* 2000(1 Pt 1):9–18.
7. Berguer R. Suboccipital approach to the distal vertebral artery. *J Vasc Surg.* 1999;30:344–349.
8. Shintani A, Zervas NT. Consequence of ligation of the vertebral artery. *J Neurosurg.* 1972;36:447–450.
9. Arden RL, Bahu SJ, Zuazu MA, Berguer R. Reflex sympathetic dystrophy of the face: current treatment recommendations. *Laryngoscope.* 1998;108:437–442.

INDEX

Note: Page numbers followed by *f* indicate figures.

RRS1308